Table of Contents

Copyright and Limited Release
Disclaimers
Important Note to Reader
Chapter 1
INTRODUCTION
Free Bonus Downloads
Introduction
Active Patients and Shared Decision Making
Medical Errors
Evidence-Based Medicine
Health Information on the Internet
Book Organization and Scope
Chapter 2
BACKGROUND & DEFINITIONS
NCI Dictionary of Cancer Terms
NCI Drug Dictionary
NCI Thesaurus
NCI Metathesaurus
Controlled Vocabularies in Health
Medical Subject Headings (MeSH)
Whiplash Journal Articles
Whiplash Internet Articles and Research
Chapter 3
EPIDEMIOLOGY
Morbidity and Disease
Sources of Morbidity Statistics
Mortality and Disease
Sources of Mortality Statistics
Whiplash Journal Articles
Whiplash Internet Articles and Research
Chapter 4
RISK FACTORS & CAUSES
Risk Factors for Disease
Causes of Disease

Whiplash Journal Articles
Whiplash Internet Articles and Research
Chapter 5
SYMPTOMS & SIGNS
Distinguishing Symtoms from Signs
Types of Symptoms
Whiplash Journal Articles
Whiplash Internet Articles and Research
Chapter 6
DIAGNOSIS
The Diagnostic and Differential Diagnostic Process
Whiplash Journal Articles
Whiplash Internet Articles and Research
Chapter 7
PATHOPHYSIOLOGY
Understanding Pathophysiology
Whiplash Journal Articles
Whiplash Internet Articles and Research
Chapter 8
TREATMENT
Treatment and Therapy
Whiplash Journal Articles
Whiplash Internet Articles and Research
Chapter 9
PROGNOSIS
Defining Prognosis
Whiplash Journal Articles
Whiplash Internet Articles and Research
Chapter 10
APPLIED RESEARCH & RESOURCES
Alternative Health & Complementary Medicine
National Center for Complementary and Alternative Medicine (NCCAM)
Nutrition
National Institutes of Health Office of Dietary Supplements (ODS)
Biotechnology & Patents
Patent Information Online
Clinical Guidelines

Agency for Healthcare Research and Quality (AHRQ)
Drugs & Medications
Prescription and Over-the-Counter Drugs and Medications
Books
National Library of Medicine's Bookshelf
Journals
MEDLINE Journals - The Abridged Index Medicus (AIM)
All MEDLINE Journals
Current Journals
Current and Previously Indexed Journals
Using Filters to Search
Journal Articles
Types of Research Articles
The National Library of Medicine
National Library of Medicine Databases
MEDLINE
PubMed
PubMed Central
PubMed Journal Citations
PubMed Central (PMC) Journal Citations
FREE EBOOK DOWNLOADS
REFERENCES

Emily Ann Davis

The Truth About...
HERBAL CURES

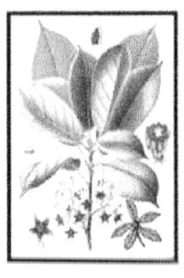

What Works...What Doesn't
The Claims & Science
Behind 46 Popular
Herbal Remedies

The Truth About Herbal Cures (106 pages)

Introduction

Broadly speaking, this book and the other volumes in this series are about health literacy. More specifically this book is about understanding the basic medical components and physiological nuance of your health condition (signs, symptoms, treatment, prognosis, etc.), researching and identifying the most authoritative and reliable information given your unique health needs (i.e. medical/physical/emotional circumstances), synthesizing this knowledge into a coherent whole, and applying your knowledge to your daily healthy living regime, or to the care of your patient or loved one.

Since this book is fundamentally about both the process and techniques involved in researching the characteristics of Whiplash and providing high quality bibliographic references about this condition, it is ideal for both the patient and the student of medicine and the life sciences, as well as others in need of authoritative, valid, and sound health information. U.S. government health experts define health literacy as "the degree to which an individual has the capacity to obtain, communicate, process, and understand basic health information and services to make appropriate health decisions." Experts agree that more than half of the adult population in the U.S. can be termed "health illiterate" and that 9 out of 10 adults are unable to understand and correctly apply even the most basic health instructions recommended by a doctor or other health care professionals. The result is that 90 million Americans are unable to take even the most basic steps to prevent disease and manage their own health conditions. Sadly, the deficiency of health knowledge is not limited to the U.S., but is widespread worldwide. This lack of health literacy, or "health illiteracy," has serious consequences; including increases in preventable deaths, increases in personal health care costs, and poor health outcomes for a majority of adults and their children.

Active Patients and Shared Decision Making

Research has demonstrated that patients who take an active role in their medical care maintain more healthy lives, recover more quickly from illness and disease, and live longer. In addition to improving health outcomes, patients who actively participate in medical decision making report increased satisfaction with their treatment, their doctors, and the health care system in general. Research has further shown that more than half of all patients are dissatisfied with the role they play in making decisions about their own personal health care.

Rather than taking a passive or subordinate role in health care, active patients partner with doctors, nurses, specialists, and other health care professionals by assuming a leadership role in managing their personal health care. These patients schedule routine medical visits, follow through on doctor recommendations and, equally as important, stay informed about health trends and health conditions that impact them. By becoming educated, these patients take the personal responsibility to learn about disease and disorders, follow evidence-based medical guidelines communicated to them by health care professionals, and strive to become knowledgeable enough to find, understand, and follow the best and most current information about illness and chronic disease management.

Because of the overall benefits of active participation in health care decision making by patients, a new health care delivery paradigm known as Shared Decision Making, or SDM, is being advocated by hospitals, researchers, and patient advocacy groups worldwide. In study after study, research has consistently and conclusively demonstrated the effectiveness of this health care model in medical disciplines ranging from preventative care, to chronic disease management (such as diabetes), to pain management, and beyond. Moreover, studies have concluded that SDM is especially effective in combating the most deadly health conditions, including the screening and treatment of cancer and heart disease.

To become an active patient, it is critical that you first know where to find reliable health information and then understand how to apply this information to your own lifestyle, health conditions, and unique set of values and personal beliefs.

This, however, isn't always as simple as it sounds. Routinely, a patient's primary (if not only) resource for medical information is the World Wide Web. Unregulated and saturated with unscrupulous "charlatans," much of the health-related information on the Web is not only inaccurate but potentially dangerous and even life-threatening. Moreover, just as technological innovation has opened up Web publishing to anyone with a network connection and a little extra time, new self-publishing platforms are making it likewise as easy for these same people to publish important looking books, regardless of the author's credentials or expertise. It is for these reasons that this book has been written with one over-arching goal in mind, to give all patients the tools and resources to become "active" patients in the care and treatment of their particular disease, disorder, or other health condition.

However, becoming an active, informed patient is only half the equation. The other half involves holding health care professionals to this same high standard of knowledge. Today physicians, nurses, and other health care professionals face numerous challenges in keeping abreast of the latest research in illness and disease and current and appropriate clinical guidelines for delivering high quality health care to patients. Popular news is replete with stories of the "crisis" in health care caused by the diminishing number of medical students choosing careers in primary care and instead opting for more lucrative specializations such as orthopedic surgery, cardiology, gastroenterology, urology, dermatology, or radiology. The result is that fewer primary care physicians are seeing more patients, spending less time with each patient, and treating more ailments, all the while struggling to manage larger caseloads and having virtually no time to stay informed on the most critical research concerning the myriad of health conditions they treat on a daily basis.

Coupled with overburdened primary care physicians, health care delivery writ large has become increasingly fragmented and it is this fragmentation that has contributed to more and more medical errors as doctors fail to adequately diagnose and communicate life-threatening conditions to both patients and other members of the health care team responsible for patient care. In 1970, the American Board of Medical Specialties (ABMS) issued certificates in only 10 medical specialties and sub-specialties. Less than 20 years later this number increased to 66 and today approximately 145 medical specialties and sub-specialties are recognized by the ABMS. The consequence is that instead of seeing one or two doctors for a particular ailment, a patient may now see four or five different physicians and specialists to treat the same condition. While all this specialization can have a positive impact on patient health, this will only be true when each member of the health care team adequately and accurately communicates test results, patient observations, and other important medical information to all the other members of the team. When communication is lacking and information is not made available to the entire team, the consequences to the patient can be catastrophic, or even life-threatening in some instances.

Finally, in America the recent expansion of the number of persons seeking and receiving health care as a result of the Affordable Care Act (ACA or "Obamacare") has overwhelmed a system already bursting at its resource seams, resulting in still more patients seeking more care from the already stressed health care system. For many of the more than eight (8) million new ACA patients, this is the first time in their lives they have had access to routine health care, including periodic check-ups, preventative care, and other basic health services. Due to the poor health care histories for these individuals and in contrast to the average patient in the pre-ACA health care population, this new group of patients is likely to enter the system with more chronic health conditions like diabetes, obesity, and high blood pressure (conditions that could have been prevented if they only had access to health care earlier). Therefore, while the ACA has increased the number of new patients by only about 3%, from approximately 256 million patients to 264 million patients, per capita it is anticipated that these patients will require more health care services than the existing patient population.

Given our beleaguered and disjointed health care system, it is no wonder that physicians and other health care professionals have virtually no time and even less energy to adequately stay informed on the most recent developments in their field. Furthermore, the sheer amount of new health information available today is immense, doubling in volume once every five (5) years. Advances in science (most notably in the study of human DNA and progress made in identifying and mapping all genes in the human genome) and technology (such as the ability to manipulate massive amounts of study data in near real-time) has rapidly increased the rate of medical advancement and made seemingly new medical innovations quickly obsolete. The cumulative effect is some doctors basing important medical decisions on outdated medical guidelines and best practices.

Because of the current state of affairs, this book is also for the health care professional. Using the same resources for patients and health professionals the goal of this book is twofold. First, this book will identify the best books, journals, journal articles, and Web resources about Whiplash available to the patient and the health care provider, therefore giving the reader a quick inventory of current research and a convenient reference during times when performing firsthand research is simply not practical, such as during a patient's appointment with her doctor. Second, it explains the most basic "mechanics" of health research and how to find and use the most trustworthy and comprehensive health care journals, databases, books, and electronic resources available in the world today. In this regard, the author hopes that this book empowers both the patient and health care professional by making each a more informed, educated, and responsible user of timely and cutting edge health information.

Though not its primary purpose, this book is in some respects a do-it-yourself guide to health-related research and resources and, as such, it is important to note this book is not prescriptive; meaning that while this book does identify limited information about causes or risk factors of Whiplash, recommend diagnostic or treatment procedures, etc., this is NOT the primary purpose of this book. Instead, this book should be used as a tool for the reader to explore and find information about Whiplash on her or his own based on their specific circumstances as patient, loved one, health care professional, researcher, or public policy-maker; keeping foremost in mind the needs and value-systems of the patient. Since health information is constantly updated and rapid medical innovation the rule rather than the exception, the author hopes this volume is not used once and forgotten to collect dust on the bookshelf, but continually and routinely referred to in order to stay abreast on the latest medical developments and apply the most recent best practices over the long-term.

Further, for patients or other "lay-persons" using this reference it is vital to understand that the knowledge gained by applying the recommendations and practices found in this book do not replace the advice and recommendations of your physician. Instead, in the spirit of SDM, the research gathered from methods used in this book should be shared with your physician and health care team to collectively determine the best course of action for a health condition keeping foremost in your specific circumstances and needs.

Finally, the author recognizes that the value of this book is based less on its content and more on its application to real-world health questions. It is therefore expected that a patient or a patient's loved one will find different utility in its pages than a health care professional. For the former, it is the author's hope that this book reduces the mystery surrounding scientific medical research and empowers the patient through knowledge and confident health care decision making. For the latter, and particularly the more highly educated health care professional, some of this material may be remedial and some simply a refresher of things you once knew but have forgotten. Since this book has also been written for the student researcher, it is the hope that this edition proves to be a valuable introduction to researching Whiplash and studying disease and health conditions in general.

Medical Errors

If you're a patient or have a loved-one receiving medical treatment and are still not convinced about the importance about being active in your health care treatment consider a 2013 article entitled *A New, Evidence-based Estimate of Patient Harms Associated with Hospital Care*, authored by John T. James, PhD, and published in the well-regarded Journal of Patient Safety. In this research article Dr. James estimates that between 210,000 and 440,000 patients die each year from preventable medical errors. If these estimates are accurate, then medical errors are the third leading cause of death in America, behind only heart disease and cancer. Similarly, other health care data suggests that 17% of all deaths in America each year can attributed to medical errors. What's as disturbing, is that these estimates only include medical errors resulting in death and do not include other harmful consequences of preventable medical errors; including permanent physical or biological damage to the patient, longer periods of hospitalization, and a lower overall quality of life. Many experts agree that if these secondary consequences of medical errors were considered the true devastation caused by medical errors would be significantly higher.

Reinforcing James' findings, another report, this one by the Office of the Inspector General for Department of Health and Human Services, studied patient care for individuals on Medicare. This 2010 study concluded that 180,000 **Medicare-only** patients die each year as a result of poor hospital care.

In his study, Dr. James cites five (5) types of preventable medical errors: errors of commission, errors of omission, errors of communication, errors of context, and diagnostic errors. **Errors of commission** occur when a health professional administers a procedure that was either performed improperly or should not have been performed at all. On the other hand **errors of omission** simply means that, based on the best medical evidence, a procedure that should have been administered, wasn't performed at all. **Communication errors** occur between two or more health professionals or between health professionals and a patient and, as the name implies, happen when critical information is not shared with members of the health care team or the patient. Communication errors can lead to a misunderstanding by medical staff as to the correct patient diagnosis or prescribed treatment regime or cause a patient to unintentionally engage in activities that are contrary to acceptable established medical recommendations for their particular disease or disorder. Similarly, **errors of context** occur when a health professional fails to consider the unique circumstances of a patient in their "post-discharge" treatment. The example used by James is the patient who lacks the mental capacity to follow an ongoing, complex treatment plan or the patient who does not have access to follow-up medical care due to financial or geographical restrictions. Finally, **diagnostic errors** occur when the incorrect diagnosis is given to a patient. Diagnosis errors often result in inappropriate treatment, ineffective treatment, and a delay in the administration of the correct treatment.

Given the troubling prevalence of medical errors, it is obvious that current diagnostic and treatment shortcomings in our health care delivery system have very real, frequently deadly implications, for the unenlightened patient and the ill-informed health care professional. Thus, it is no exaggeration to strongly caution the uninformed, un-involved patient to proceed at her own risk.

Evidence-Based Medicine

Evidence-based medicine is currently the most widely accepted and applied model of patient care in Western medicine. The most commonly accepted definition of evidence-based (EBM) medicine is one offered by Dr. David Sackett who defines EBM as "the conscientious, explicit and judicious use of current best evidence in making decisions about the care of the individual patient. It means integrating individual clinical expertise with the best available external clinical evidence from systematic research."(Sackett, Rosenberg, Gray, Haynes, & Richardson, 1996).

Therefore, EBM is the integration of the best medical evidence, as found through literature reviews and research, the clinical expertise and experience of the doctor, and a constant recognition of patient values and concerns. Fundamental to the EBM model is its reliance on research and literature reviews to give the doctor and patient the best possible benchmark or baseline information to begin to answer relevant clinical questions and formulate a treatment plan both appropriate and acceptable to the patient. It is the goal of this book to provide the reader with both the basic medical literature research tools, as well as a bibliography of some of the important research itself. However, it is important to remember that even though evidence and research are primary in the EBM decision making process, it is not the sole deciding factor in determining patient care and on a case-by-case basis may in some instances not even be the most important consideration.

The EBM process begins by identifying a clinical problem and then applying this problem to a specific question about treating and caring for the individual patient. Based on the question, the doctor or researcher then determines the best available resource or resources to answer that question. Next, the literature is reviewed keeping in mind two important questions. First, is the literature **valid**, meaning does it accurately represent the truth as we know it today and does it have a sound basis in reason and fact. Second, does the literature offer advice and recommendations that are **applicable** to the patient and therefore will, if followed, offer a reasonable expectation of a successful patient outcome. Once the doctor has made her evaluation and formed a recommendation or alternative recommendations, she presents her conclusions and recommendations to the patient and in consult together they examine the evidence and discuss the patient's preferences and values to agree on a course of medical treatment.

Health Information on the Internet

Since most disease and health-related information is accessed by both patients and medical professionals via the Internet, either through general queries using search engines like Google or by directly accessing professional databases and information repositories, it is important be able to determine what constitutes quality health information. A 2013 survey by the Pew Research Center found that "59% of U.S. adults have looked online for information about a range of health related topics in the past year", and "35% of U.S. adults say they have gone online specifically to try to figure out what medical condition they or someone else might have." While the Internet can be a quality resource to find information quickly and easily, there are many important questions to answer to evaluate the information you find online, such as:

Which websites and databases are most reliable?

How do you analyze the information you've found?

How current is the information you've found?

Unfortunately, not everyone reading this book is a medical professional and everyone doesn't possess the same background or knowledge base to understand and filter all the information found online. This section will therefore examine some factors to consider when evaluating health information on the Internet.

More often than not, your first foray into researching all but the most basic health information online will end in confusion. While there is no shortage of health information on the Internet, at best much of what you will find will consist of over-generalizations of complex conditions, and analysis and recommendations not tailored to your specific concerns. At worst some of the information you find online will be founded upon baseless scientific conclusions, and downright dangerous home remedies. Certainly, your first rule of thumb needs to be that under no circumstance should you trust the veracity of everything written online. To make sense of what you find it is critical to keep a number of questions in mind prior to acting on any online health advice:

First, consider the source.

Look for an "about us" page. What is the original source of the information and what are the credentials of the person or organization that provided it? This information could be very telling.

Notice whether or not the website providing health related information shares its source(s)? If it does, is it a reliable source? Remember, much (if not most) information posted on websites actually originates from a third-party source. If the organization or person that owns or administers the website did not author the content the actual source should be conspicuously identified. Also, if the information wasn't written by a medical expert, was the information reviewed and approved for quality by an expert with professional credentials in that field?

If a non-medical person or organization wrote the article is it reliable? You should limit your research to only reliable sources. A reliable source could include websites published published by the U.S. government, non-for-profit entities, and universities or other institutions of higher learning. Respectively, these websites can be identified with dot gov, dot org or dot edu URL extensions. Does information on the website appear to be more opinion than fact? If it is opinion-based, does it come from a an expert area of study or unbiased and objective organization such as a medical association or research institute? These sites are generally the most trustworty as they are not affiliated with insurance or pharmaceutical companies, and therefore have no profit-based motive (or appearance of one) in providing certain conclusions or advice. Having said that, it is still recommended you to dig deeper to discover exactly where the information originated.

Today, most web search engines like Google make it easy to limit your searches to .org or .gov websites. Simply type in your search term (enclosed in quotations for multiple words) followed by "site:.org" or "site:.gov" without the quotations here of course. Always remember to include the dot after the colon in "site."

For example, to search the broad topic of Whiplash simply type:

"Whiplash" site:.org

or

"Whiplash" site:.gov

Domain names with the .com web extension generally represent businesses or other for profit companies. Business websites have the primary purpose of selling products or services, instead of providing reliable health information. If this is the case, the health information could be skewed to make their product or service more appealing.

While commercial sites **may** offer some useful and accurate information you will want to remain vigilant and be sure to cross-check any of the information you find with a more reliable source. While it is possible that the information can be trusted, if it seems to be provided only to make a certain product or service more appealing it is best to be skeptical and move on to the next resource.

Finally, a third source of online information is websites published by individuals. Many of these sites offer support and advice about coping with certain conditions and their treatments. While these websites can contain reliable and useful information, it is necessarily biased by only one person's experience. Additionally, diseases and health conditions impact different people differently and there are numerous factors that need to be considered before relying wholesale on one person's experience. These factors may be demographic, such as age or gender, physical, including the person's overall health or other aggravating health conditions, or even the quality of health care the individual received.

Second, how current is the information?

Rapid advances in research means health information is continually changing. Daily, research discoveries and advancements change the landscapes in our understanding of countless diseases. As such, it is critical that a website clearly idenifies the date it was last updated. Most reliable web pages will include information about when the information was last updated or reviewed, in addition to a statement about how information is reviewed to stay current. The date is usually located towards the end of an article. If no date is posted, located the copyright notice. This will tell you the date the article was originally published or written and the publishing organization, if applicable. If the article is more than a year or two old, you are likely better off finding more current information.

Third, does the site present facts and not opinion?

Information should be clearly written, based in fact and present the full scope of the issue being studied, and not just selective anecdotes. The content should be easily verified from a trustworthy information source such as professional journal articles, abstracts, or doctors and other medical professionals.

Fourth, who is the intended audience?

It should be clearly stated on the website whether the information is intended for the consumer, or the health professional. Many websites have separate web pages for patients and doctors or health care professionals. Be sure to use the information that is most relevant to your information needs.

Fifth, be skeptical.

Claims that sound too good to be true often are. Your goal should be to find current, unbiased information based on scientifically valid research. If you're a patient, it is important to remember that no matter how confident you are in your online research it can not replace the advice of your doctor, as she is most familiar with your specific medical circumstances. Your doctor is the best person to answer questions about your personal health. She not only understands your health history and any medication you take, she also understands the plethora of other health factors that may be involved and interact and she's committed to providing the best possible care and treatment.

Book Organization and Scope

This book begins by providing the reader with background information and definitions related to Whiplash. Importantly, the second chapter also identifies and explains specific high-quality resources the reader can trust when performing individual health research on specific topics and sub-topics. Chapters 3 through 9 proceed to discuss the individual components of *all* health-related conditions, including epidemiology, risk factors and cause, signs and symptoms, diagnosis, pathophysiology, treatment, and prognosis. Importantly, each of these chapters begin by explaining precisely what is a meant by a doctor when she discusses each of these concepts and ends with an examination of how each applies to the medical condition of Whiplash. While this book focuses on the "nut-and-bolts" of Whiplash, Chapter 10 concludes by providing the the interested reader with additional resources to expand their research to other areas, including but not limited to the role nutrition in preventing or treating Whiplash, alternative therapies, and biotechnology.

Importantly, as a research reference, throughout this book hundreds of articles are identified to enable the reader examine particular issues in depth. Each list of references contains a wide assortment of articles and includes research studies and articles geared towards readers of all levels of sophistication, from research novices and patients to and medical and health-care professionals. Each article is hyperlinked directly to the source allowing the reader to access without leaving the book. Additionally, each reference is linked directly and not hidden beneath confusing anchor text thereby allowing the reader to identify the precise source and location of the article for further future reference.

While this book is organized in a manner that most closely resembles the order of disease or disorder progression, from pre-disability considerations to symptoms, treatment, and eventual outcome, it is first and foremost a reference book. This means a reader can read chapters and sections in isolation and without first reading a preceding chapter or section, as the entire book is written in a manner making it easy for the reader to refer to areas of immediate interest without fear of losing meaning or nuance that may have been discussed earlier in the book.

CHAPTER 2
BACKGROUND
&
DEFINITIONS

The purpose of this chapter is to provide the reader with resources to find high-level definitions of terminology associated with Whiplash. The easiest way to begin your understanding of complex health concepts is to first understand the definitions of key words and phrases commonly associated with a disease or illness. It is helpful to look up the words you are unfamiliar with, and keep a list of definitions for your reference. Often, a common term in a non-scientific context has a completely different meaning than the same term has in medicine, so be prepared to investigate and find words that are more familiar to you if you cannot understand a term or make the standard definition work in your particular context. As you become more familiar with your topic, the vocabulary will become less daunting and difficult ideas will be more understandable. Once you have a grasp of the content of your research, spend some time thinking about the research. Critically interpret what the results mean and how they are relevant to the disease. Keep in mind that in contrast to words used in everyday writing or conversation, scientific and medical terms have very precise meanings. In this regard, you will frequently encounter two or more medical terms that *seem* to have identical meanings, only to discover later that the distinction between these terms is critically important in a medical context.

This chapter will first identify the best sources for finding reliable definitions and explanations for complex health and medical terms and introduce the concept of a "controlled vocabularly." This chapter will conclude with definitions of the most commonly used terms associated with Whiplash.

NCI Dictionary of Cancer Terms

The *National Cancer Institute (NCI) Dictionary of Cancer Terms* contains definition and information for 7,665 medical terms. While developed and hosted by the NCI, the dictionary contains definitions for both cancer- and non-cancer-related medical concepts. To search, simply type in your search term and click the **go** button. To find all words in the dictionary that include your search term, click the radio button **Contains** and all definitions with your search term will be available. For example, searching the term "thyroid" will return results for 28 terms containing the word "thyroid" including "anaplastic thyroid cancer" "autoimmune thyroiditis," "familial isolated hyperparathyroidism," etc. You can also select the letter your term begins with and scroll to the term you are looking up. The search box contains an **autosuggest** feature so after you type in the first three letters of the word, you will be presented with the first 10 terms that begin with those letters. If your word doesn't appear within the first 10 suggestions simply continue to type in additional letters and eventually the dictionary will narrow its suggestions to the term you need. This is particularly helpful for longer terms and words difficult to spell. If you want to turn the autosuggest feature off simply hit escape or click **close** within the autosuggest box. The results include the definition for your selected terms as well as a pronunciation guide. If you want to hear how the word sounds, simply click the audio radio icon button next to the term name. The NCI Dictionary of Cancer Terms can be accessed at: http://www.cancer.gov/dictionary

NCI Drug Dictionary

The NCI Drug Dictionary defines terms and alternative research links for medications and drug agents used for cancer theryapy, as well as countless other health conditions. The search engine operates in a manner identical to the one used by the NCI Dictionary of Cancer Terms so the same tips apply. All definitions include synonyms and generic and brand names for the drug. One excellent feature of the the NCI Drug Dictionary is that it also includes links to both open and closed clinical research trials related to that medication. The NCI Drug Dictionary can be found at: http://www.cancer.gov/drugdictionary

NCI Thesaurus

The NCI Thesaurus (NCIt) is a database of reference terms for many health-related from the NCI and other health databases.

The NCIt is updated frequently by a team of medical experts and contains more than 200,000 links and cross-references to other research information related to your term. Most people believe that a thesaurus is used only to identify synonyms for individual words or phrases. This is not totally correct as the more important purpose of a good thesaurus is to identify related concepts and ideas. In this regard the NCI Thesaurus and the NCI Metathesaurus (discussed below) are wonderful resources to reference when defining terms and determining the scope of your information needs.

The thesaurus can be searched at: http://ncit.nci.nih.gov.

If you prefer to work offline, the entire thesaurus can also be downloaded at: http://evs.nci.nih.gov/ftp1/NCI_Thesaurus.

NCI Metathesaurus

The NCI Metathesaurus (NCIm) is a vast medical research terminology database that provides definition and conceptual information for more than 4 million terms related to clinical care, biomedical research, and health care administration in general. The NCIm also has more than 22 million links and cross-references to additional concepts and information related to health and disease. To search the NCIm simply go to: http://ncim.nci.nih.gov/ncimbrowser.

Controlled Vocabularies in Health

The single most important purpose of a controlled vocabulary is to make searching a database easier. The Library Archives of Canada defines a controlled vocabulary as an "established list of standardized terminology for use in indexing and retrieval of information." Controlled vocabularies are used to capture, store, organize, search, analyze, and normalize information allowing for the exchange of information across different platforms.

While the term controlled vocabulary may seem foreign, you are likely already familiar with applications of the concept of in other contexts. Using a series of cross-references, the Yellow Page listings in a telephone book use a controlled vocabulary to make searching for specific types of businesses or organizations easier. For example, a Yellow Page search for "Doctors" doesn't list doctors at all but instead says "*see* Chiropractors; Physicians - MD & DO; Podiatrists; Psychologists" thereby directing the reader to search for a doctor or type of doctor under these headings instead. This alternative listing for "Doctors" is a controlled vocabulary and like all controlled vocabularies serves three very important purposes.

The first is to keep the size of a database manageable. Imagine the amount of needless repetition that would occur if under the heading "Doctors" a complete listing of doctors was shown and the identical list appeared again under the subject heading "Physicians - MD & DO." Consider then the additional clutter created for duplicate listings for "Cars" and "Automobiles," "Grocery" and "Supermarkets," "Churches" and "Worship Services," "Job Services," and "Employment" and on and on. If this were done, it wouldn't take long for the size of the Yellow Pages in even communities of modest size to exceed that of a complete set of the old Encyclopedia Britannica. This concept of managing the size of information also holds true for computerized databases where the space needed to store duplicate entries is prohibitive in terms of bandwidth and storage costs.

The second, and more important purpose of the controlled vocabulary, is to make your search more efficient and more precise. Using our Yellow Pages example, imagine if a search under the term "Doctor" yielded nothing and the term itself wasn't even listed and you were expected to know to look under "Physicians - MD & DO" instead. While many people may have the wherewithal to look to the "Physician" listing this may not be true for people looking for contact information for businesses or organization in more esoteric fields. Thus, the controlled vocabulary makes it easy to find what you need by essentially saying "you're close, good try but go here instead and you will find exactly what you need."

Finally, controlled vocabularies make complex topics like medicine accessible to novices and other non-subject-matter-expert researchers. Have you ever had a rough concept of what you were you trying to locate but either didn't know its precise term or were unable to recall it? In instances like this a controlled vocabulary can be indispensable allowing you to enter a term close to the one needed but not exact and then returning a list of related concepts and terms where one is likely to meet your precise needs. In this way, a controlled vocabulary acts like a thesaurus of words or phrases. While some believe a thesaurus returns a list of exact synonyms for a chosen word, in truth the meanings for words in a thesaurus are most often similar but not exact. Therefore, when searching a thesaurus you really aren't trying to find a *fancier* word with the same meaning but a word that most precisely communicates the the idea you are attempting to convey in terms of meaning, magnitude, or degree.

In the online world, most websites and databases that store large sets of information incorporate at least a basic form controlled vocabularies. If you are familiar with the online concept of "keyword tagging" (like the use of the hash tag "#" in twitter "tweets" to affiliate messages with other message on the same topic), this is exactly what controlled vocabularies attempt to accomplish, albeit in a more sophisticated and organized manner. Like keyword tagging, establishing a controlled vocabulary is not a one-time endeavor, but a constant and ongoing exercise where categories and search words and phrases are updated continuously to accommodate new terms, ideas, and discoveries.

In the age of technology, it is important to point out that contrary to our Yellow Pages example the use of controlled vocabulary today is almost exclusively the province of the Internet. In Health and Medicine, the international gold standard of controlled vocabularies is known as MeSH, or Medical Subject Headings. MeSH is discussed further below.

Medical Subject Headings (MeSH)

MeSH or Medical Subject Headings is the U.S. National Library of Medicine's thesaurus. Use MeSH as a starting point for your research to collect relevant keywords and terms for further searches in the databases discussed later in this book. Since MeSH is both a controlled vocabulary and thesaurus the terms that appear in a MeSH search also include term definitions. These definitions should be recorded together with the MeSH search terms. Use MeSH definitions to understand important concepts and MeSH terms to establish a list of keywords for more in-depth and precise research.

MeSH is used by the NLM to catalogue all MEDLINE and PubMED

databases, as well as NLM database of documents, books, and video and other NLM holdings. MeSH can be accessed by going to http://www.ncbi.nlm.nih.gov/mesh.

Whiplash Journal Articles

Banic, B., Petersen-Felix, S., Andersen, O. K., Radanov, B. P., Villiger, P. M., Arendt-Nielsen, L., & Curatolo, M. (2004). Evidence for spinal cord hypersensitivity in chronic pain after whiplash injury and in fibromyalgia. *Pain, 107*(1-2), 7–15. http://doi.org/10.1016/j.pain.2003.05.001

Bannister, G., Amirfeyz, R., Kelley, S., & Gargan, M. (2009). Whiplash injury. *The Journal of Bone and Joint Surgery. British Volume, 91*(7), 845–850. http://doi.org/10.1302/0301-620X.91B7.22639

Barnsley, L., Lord, S., & Bogduk, N. (1994). Whiplash injury. *Pain, 58*(3), 283–307.

Chen, H., Yang, K. H., & Wang, Z. (2009). Biomechanics of whiplash injury. *Chinese Journal of Traumatology = Zhonghua Chuang Shang Za Zhi / Chinese Medical Association, 12*(5), 305–314. http://doi.org/10.3760/cma.j.issn.1008-1275.2009.05.011

Chien, A., Eliav, E., & Sterling, M. (2009). Hypoaesthesia occurs with sensory hypersensitivity in chronic whiplash - Further evidence of a neuropathic condition. *Manual Therapy, 14*(2), 138–146. http://doi.org/10.1016/j.math.2007.12.004

Cholewicki, J., Panjabi, M. M., Nibu, K., Babat, L. B., Grauer, J. N., & Dvorak, J. (1998). Head kinematics during in vitro whiplash simulation. *Accident Analysis and Prevention, 30*(4), 469–479. http://doi.org/10.1016/S0001-4575(97)00103-6

Côté, P., Cassidy, J. D., Carroll, L., Frank, J. W., & Bombardier, C. (2001). A systematic review of the prognosis of acute whiplash and a new conceptual framework to synthesize the literature. *Spine, 26*(19), E445–E458. http://doi.org/10.1097/00007632-200110010-00020

Daenen, L., Nijs, J., Raadsen, B., Roussel, N., Cras, P., & Dankaerts, W. (2013). Cervical motor dysfunction and its predictive value for long-term recovery in patients with acute whiplash-associated disorders: a systematic review. *Journal of Rehabilitation Medicine : Official Journal of the UEMS*

European Board of Physical and Rehabilitation Medicine, *45*(2), 113–22. http://doi.org/10.2340/16501977-1091

Dall'Alba, P. T., Sterling, M. M., Treleaven, J. M., Edwards, S. L., & Jull, G. A. (2001). Cervical range of motion discriminates between asymptomatic persons and those with whiplash. *Spine*, *26*(19), 2090–2094. http://doi.org/10.1097/00007632-200110010-00009

Davis, C. G. (2013). Mechanisms of chronic pain from whiplash injury. *Journal of Forensic and Legal Medicine*. http://doi.org/10.1016/j.jflm.2012.05.004

Dommerholt, J. (2005). Persistent myalgia following whiplash. *Current Pain and Headache Reports*, *9*(5), 326–330. http://doi.org/10.1007/s11916-005-0008-5

Elliott, J. M., Noteboom, J. T., Flynn, T. W., & Sterling, M. (2009). Characterization of acute and chronic whiplash-associated disorders. *The Journal of Orthopaedic and Sports Physical Therapy*, *39*(5), 312–323. http://doi.org/10.2519/jospt.2009.2826

Endo, K., Ichimaru, K., Komagata, M., & Yamamoto, K. (2006). Cervical vertigo and dizziness after whiplash injury. *European Spine Journal*, *15*(6), 886–890. http://doi.org/10.1007/s00586-005-0970-y

Fernández De Las Peñas, C., Palomeque Del Cerro, L., & Fernández Carnero, J. (2005). Manual treatment of post-whiplash injury. *Journal of Bodywork and Movement Therapies*, *9*(2), 109–119. http://doi.org/10.1016/j.jbmt.2004.05.002

Ferrari, R. (2003). Myths of whiplash. *The Surgeon : Journal of the Royal Colleges of Surgeons of Edinburgh and Ireland*, *1*(2), 99, 101–103. http://doi.org/10.1016/S1479-666X(03)80124-5

Ferrari, R. (2010). Predicting central sensitisation: Whiplash patients. *Australian Family Physician*, *39*(11), 863–866.

Freeman, M. D., Croft, A. C., & Rossignol, A. M. (1998). "Whiplash associated disorders: redefining whiplash and its management" by the Quebec Task Force. A critical evaluation. *Spine, 23*(9), 1043–1049. http://doi.org/10.1097/00007632-199805010-00015

Haneline, M. T. (2009). The notion of a "whiplash culture": a review of the evidence. *Journal of Chiropractic Medicine*. http://doi.org/10.1016/j.jcm.2009.04.001

Ito, S., Panjabi, M. M., Ivancic, P. C., & Pearson, A. M. (2004). Spinal canal narrowing during simulated whiplash. *Spine, 29*(12), 1330–1339. http://doi.org/10.1097/01.BRS.0000127186.81814.4A

Ivancic, P. C., Ito, S., Tominaga, Y., Rubin, W., Coe, M. P., Ndu, A. B., … Panjabi, M. M. (2008). Whiplash causes increased laxity of cervical capsular ligament. *Clinical Biomechanics, 23*(2), 159–165. http://doi.org/10.1016/j.clinbiomech.2007.09.003

Ivancic, P. C., Panjabi, M. M., Ito, S., Cripton, P. A., & Wang, J. L. (2005). Biofidelic whole cervical spine model with muscle force replication for whiplash simulation. *European Spine Journal, 14*(4), 346–355. http://doi.org/10.1007/s00586-004-0758-5

Jull, G. A., Söderlund, A., Stemper, B. D., Kenardy, J., Gross, A. R., Côté, P., … Curatolo, M. (2011). Toward Optimal Early Management After Whiplash Injury to Lessen the Rate of Transition to Chronicity. *Spine*. http://doi.org/10.1097/BRS.0b013e3182388449

Jull, G., Kristjansson, E., & Dall'Alba, P. (2004). Impairment in the cervical flexors: A comparison of whiplash and insidious onset neck pain patients. *Manual Therapy, 9*(2), 89–94. http://doi.org/10.1016/S1356-689X(03)00086-9

Klein, G. N., Mannion, A. F., Panjabi, M. M., & Dvorak, J. (2001). Trapped in the neutral zone: Another symptom of whiplash-associated disorder? *European Spine Journal, 10*(2), 141–148. http://doi.org/10.1007/s005860100248

Krakenes, J., & Kaale, B. R. (2006). Magnetic resonance imaging assessment of craniovertebral ligaments and membranes after whiplash trauma. *Spine*, *31*(24), 2820–2826. http://doi.org/10.1097/01.brs.0000245871.15696.1f

Kumar, S., Ferrari, R., & Narayan, Y. (2005). Kinematic and electromyographic response to whiplash loading in low-velocity whiplash impacts - A review. *Clinical Biomechanics*. http://doi.org/10.1016/j.clinbiomech.2004.11.016

Marx, P. (2011). Assessment of whiplash and cervical spine injury. *Der Nervenarzt*. http://doi.org/10.1007/s00115-011-3286-7

Mayou, R., & Bryant, B. (2002). Psychiatry of whiplash neck injury. *British Journal of Psychiatry*, *180*(MAY), 441–448. http://doi.org/10.1192/bjp.180.5.441

Panjabi, M. M., Cholewicki, J., Nibu, K., Grauer, J. N., Babat, L. B., & Dvorak, J. (1998). Mechanism of whiplash injury. *Clinical Biomechanics*, *13*(4-5), 239–249. http://doi.org/10.1016/S0268-0033(98)00033-3

Panjabi, M. M., Cholewicki, J., Nibu, K., Grauer, J. N., Babat, L. B., Dvorak, J., & Bär, H. F. (1998). Biomechanics of whiplash injury. *Der Orthopade*, *27*(12), 813–819. http://doi.org/10.3760/cma.j.issn.1008-1275.2009.05.011

Panjabi, M. M., Pearson, A. M., Ito, S., Ivancic, P. C., & Wang, J. L. (2004). Cervical spine curvature during simulated whiplash. *Clinical Biomechanics*, *19*(1), 1–9. http://doi.org/10.1016/j.clinbiomech.2003.09.006

Pinfold, M., Niere, K. R., O'Leary, E. F., Hoving, J. L., Green, S., & Buchbinder, R. (2004). Validity and internal consistency of a whiplash-specific disability measure. *Spine*, *29*(3), 263–268. http://doi.org/10.1097/01.BRS.0000107238.15526.4C

Poorbaugh, K., Brismée, J. M., Phelps, V., & Sizer, P. S. (2008). Late Whiplash Syndrome: A clinical science approach to evidence-based diagnosis and management. *Pain Practice*, *8*(1), 65–89. http://doi.org/10.1111/j.1533-2500.2007.00168.x

Rebbeck, T. J., Refshauge, K. M., Maher, C. G., & Stewart, M. (2007).

Evaluation of the core outcome measure in whiplash. *Spine*, *32*(6), 696–702. http://doi.org/10.1097/01.brs.0000257595.75367.52

Scholten-Peeters, G. G. M., Bekkering, G. E., Verhagen, A. P., van Der Windt, D. A. W. M., Lanser, K., Hendriks, E. J. M., & Oostendorp, R. A. B. (2002). Clinical practice guideline for the physiotherapy of patients with whiplash-associated disorders. *Spine*, *27*(4), 412–422. http://doi.org/10.1097/00007632-200202150-00018

Siegmund, G. P. (2011). What Occupant Kinematics and Neuromuscular Responses Tell Us About Whiplash Injury. *Spine*. http://doi.org/10.1097/BRS.0b013e3182387d71

Siegmund, G. P., Winkelstein, B. A., Ivancic, P. C., Svensson, M. Y., & Vasavada, A. (2009). The anatomy and biomechanics of acute and chronic whiplash injury. *Traffic Injury Prevention*, *10*(2), 101–112. http://doi.org/10.1080/15389580802593269

Sizer, P. S., Poorbaugh, K., & Phelps, V. (2004). Whiplash associated disorders: pathomechanics, diagnosis, and management. *Pain Practice : The Official Journal of World Institute of Pain*, *4*(3), 249–266. http://doi.org/10.1111/j.1533-2500.2004.04310.x

Sterling, M. (2004). A proposed new classification system for whiplash associated disorders--implications for assessment and management. *Manual Therapy*, *9*(2), 60–70. http://doi.org/10.1016/j.math.2004.01.006

Sterling, M. Physical and psychological aspects of whiplash: important considerations for primary care assessment, part 2--case studies., 14 Manual therapy e8–e12 (2009). http://doi.org/10.1016/j.math.2008.03.004

Sterling, M., Jull, G., & Kenardy, J. (2006). Physical and psychological factors maintain long-term predictive capacity post-whiplash injury. *Pain*, *122*(1-2), 102–108. http://doi.org/10.1016/j.pain.2006.01.014

Sterling, M., Jull, G., Vicenzino, B., & Kenardy, J. (2004). *Characterization of acute whiplash-associated disorders. Spine* (Vol. 29).

Sterling, M., Jull, G., Vicenzino, B., Kenardy, J., & Darnell, R. (2005). Physical and psychological factors predict outcome following whiplash injury. *Pain, 114*(1-2), 141–148. http://doi.org/10.1016/j.pain.2004.12.005

Sterling, M., & Kenardy, J. (2008). Physical and psychological aspects of whiplash: Important considerations for primary care assessment. *Manual Therapy, 13*(2), 93–102. http://doi.org/10.1016/j.math.2007.11.003

Sterling, M., Treleaven, J., & Jull, G. (2002). Responses to a clinical test of mechanical provocation of nerve tissue in whiplash associated disorder. *Manual Therapy, 7*(2), 89–94. http://doi.org/10.1054/math.2002.0443

Treleaven, J., Jull, G., & Sterling, M. (2003). Dizziness and unsteadiness following whiplash injury: Characteristic features and relationship with cervical joint position error. *Journal of Rehabilitation Medicine, 35*(1), 36–43. http://doi.org/10.1080/16501970306109

Verhagen, A. P., Lewis, M., Schellingerhout, J. M., Heymans, M. W., Dziedzic, K., de Vet, H. C. W., & Koes, B. W. (2011). Do whiplash patients differ from other patients with non-specific neck pain regarding pain, function or prognosis? *Manual Therapy, 16*(5), 456–462. http://doi.org/10.1016/j.math.2011.02.009

Verhagen, A. P., Scholten-Peeters, G. G. G. M., Van Wijngaarden, S., De Bie, R. A., & Bierma-Zeinstra, S. M. A. (2007). Conservative treatments for whiplash. *Cochrane Database of Systematic Reviews*. http://doi.org/10.1002/14651858.CD003338.pub3

Yadla, S., Ratliff, J. K., & Harrop, J. S. (2008). Whiplash: Diagnosis, treatment, and associated injuries. *Current Reviews in Musculoskeletal Medicine*. http://doi.org/10.1007/s12178-007-9008-x

Yoganandan, N., Pintar, F. A., & Cusick, J. F. (2002). Biomechanical analyses of whiplash injuries using an experimental model. *Accident Analysis and Prevention, 34*(5), 663–671. http://doi.org/10.1016/S0001-4575(01)00066-5

Whiplash Internet Articles and Research

Cervical Sprain and Strain. (2015). Retrieved on February 2, 2015, from http://emedicine.medscape.com/article/306176-overview.

Curbing the whiplash epidemic | Barnett Waddingham. (2015). Retrieved on February 2, 2015, from http://www.barnett-waddingham.co.uk/comment-insight/blog/2014/11/03/curbing-whiplash-epidemic/.

Definition of "whiplash injury" | Collins English Dictionary. (2015). Retrieved on February 2, 2015, from http://www.collinsdictionary.com/dictionary/english/whiplash-injury.

Incidence of whiplash. (2015). Retrieved on February 2, 2015, from http://www.bcmj.org/article/incidence-whiplash-associated-disorder.

Sprains And Strains Cervical Spine Neck. (2015). Retrieved on February 2, 2015, from http://www.mdguidelines.com/sprains-and-strains-cervical-spine-neck.

Three Common Car Accident Injuries | by Nolo. (2015). Retrieved on February 2, 2015, from http://www.all-about-car-accidents.com/resources/auto-accident/car-accident-injuries/3-common-types-car-crash-injuries.

What is whiplash? What causes whiplash?. (2015). Retrieved on February 2, 2015, from http://www.medicalnewstoday.com/articles/174605.php.

Whiplash (medicine). (2015). Retrieved on February 2, 2015, from http://en.wikipedia.org/wiki/Whiplash_(medicine).

Whiplash Associated Disorders. (2015). Retrieved on February 2, 2015, from http://www.physio-pedia.com/Whiplash_Associated_Disorders.

Whiplash Definition. (2015). Retrieved on February 2, 2015, from http://www.mayoclinic.org/diseases-conditions/whiplash/basics/definition/con-20033090.

Whiplash Injuries: The Basics | Nolo.com. (2015). Retrieved on February 2, 2015, from http://www.nolo.com/legal-encyclopedia/whiplash-injuries-basics-32286.html.

Whiplash Injuries. (2015). Retrieved on February 2, 2015, from http://www.nfsesq.com/resources/whiplash-terminology/.

Whiplash Legal Definition. (2015). Retrieved on February 2, 2015, from http://www.duhaime.org/LegalDictionary/W/Whiplash.aspx.

Whiplash injury definition. (2015). Retrieved on February 2, 2015, from http://www.medicinenet.com/script/main/art.asp?articlekey=11605.

Whiplash | Define Whiplash at Dictionary.com. (2015). Retrieved on February 2, 2015, from http://dictionary.reference.com/browse/whiplash.

Whiplash | University of Maryland Medical Center. (2015). Retrieved on February 2, 2015, from http://umm.edu/health/medical/ency/articles/whiplash.

Whiplash. (2015). Retrieved on February 2, 2015, from http://backandneck.about.com/od/bodymechanics/a/whiplash.htm.

Whiplash. (2015). Retrieved on February 2, 2015, from http://www.nhs.uk/Conditions/Whiplash/Pages/Symptoms.aspx.

whiplash legal definition of whiplash. (2015). Retrieved on February 2, 2015, from http://legal-dictionary.thefreedictionary.com/whiplash.

whiplash. (2015). Retrieved on February 2, 2015, from http://medical-dictionary.thefreedictionary.com/whiplash.

whiplash. (2015). Retrieved on February 2, 2015, from http://www.thefreedictionary.com/whiplash.

Conlin A , et al.. (2015). *Treatment of whiplash*. Retrieved on February 2, 2015, from http://www.ncbi.nlm.nih.gov/pubmed/15782245.

Radanov BP , et al.. (2015). *Long*. Retrieved on February 2, 2015, from http://www.ncbi.nlm.nih.gov/pubmed/7565068.

CHAPTER 3
EPIDEMIOLOGY

Epidemiology is the branch of medicine concerned with researching factors related to the distribution of disease in human populations. Important components of epidemiological research include studying the cause, incidence, prevalence, behavior, and transmission of disease affecting groups of people. Epidemiology is most often associated with public health since it is primarily concerned with disease outbreaks in human populations, in contrast to disease manifestation in individuals. Depending on research needs, the population studied can be of any size and composition as long members of the group share specific characteristics important to the researcher. For instance, study populations can be based on geography, where populations as large as individual nations or entire continents are examined. Conversely, populations may be as small a remote village or a single work site where all individuals are exposed to identical environmental toxins, such as airborne coal dust inhaled by workers at a local coal mine. While geography is often an important consideration in epidemiological research, groups can also be studied based on numerous factors unrelated to physical location, such as age, gender, race or nationality, diet, and so on.

Since epidemiology and pathology both study disease, people often find it difficult to distinguish between the two scientific disciplines. One easy, albeit vastly oversimplified way to distinguish between the two disciplines, is that epidemiology is the study of disease in groups of people while pathology studies disease in an individual person or organism.

Morbidity and Disease

Two of the most basic and important concepts in Epidemiology are incidence and prevalence. Incidence and prevalence are both measures of morbidity. Quite simply, morbidity is **the extent of illness, injury or disability in a defined population**. In epidemiology, incidence and prevalence are important in that both statistics attempt to measure risk, where risk is **the likelihood that an individual within a population will contract a disease**. While both incidence and prevalence attempt to estimate the occurrence of a health condition during a specified period of time, many people confuse incidence and prevalence and use them interchangeably falsely assuming that one is simply a synonym for the other. However, when researching Whiplash it is important to remember that each term has its own distinct meaning.

The term incidence refers to the number of new cases of a health condition in a given time period. In other words, incidence most closely resembles the number of new diagnoses. Conversely, prevalence means the number of persons *currently* suffering from a health condition. In this regard, a person diagnosed with a *chronic* health condition (where *chronic* describes an illness persisting over a long time period) will be included in incidence statistics in only one year, that being the year they were diagnosed but this same individual will be included prevalence reports each year they suffer this health condition. Taken one step further, a newly diagnosed patient will be counted in both incidence and prevalence statistics during the patient's first year of a health condition but in subsequent years will only be included in prevalence statistics. The important takeaway, therefore, is that for any given timeframe the prevalance of a health condition will always be equal or greater than the incidence of the same condition. Most of the time incidence and prevalence statistics are reported on an annual basis, though for health conditions like Influenza seasonal or monthly morbidity may be more important.

Because these two concepts have distinct meanings they are most revealing taken together and often the two numbers can vary dramatically from one another. For short-lived health conditions like Influenza incidence can be very high during years with large outbreaks as large populations may suffer from a vaccine resistant Influenza strain but the overall prevalence may be quite low in subsequent years. On the other hand, for some chronic illnesses the incidence rate may be low when compared to the prevalence rate. An example is when public health researchers introduce new preventative treatment strategies for a certain health condition. Currently, enormous resources are being used to prevent Type II Diabetes. Why? Because in recent years there has been a dramatic rise in the number of individuals diagnosed with this disease, resulting in a large number of individuals managing Diabetes in any given year. However, if preventative efforts are successful we can expect the number of new diagnoses in the first "successful" year to decline dramatically. Therefore, in that year the incidence of the disease will significantly decline but those already afflicted with the disease may still keep the prevalence statistics high.

Thus, when reviewing incidence and prevalence statistics it is worthwhile to compare the figures over more than one year. If, for example, you notice that incidence and prevalence rates are both high for nine (9) consecutive years but the incidence rate drops dramatically in the tenth year you may rightly hypothesize that a new preventative treatment was introduced in the tenth year therefore leading you to research your assumption further.

It is also important to remember that incidence and prevalence statistics do not attempt to measure the entire population. Instead these statistics generally only measure populations at risk. To illustrate, incidence and prevalence measures of Cervical Cancer only include women. Likewise, Testicular Cancer is only calculated for men. While this is important to remember, the research you will discover will clearly report the population the estimate is intended to reflect.

Mathematically, with "/" meaning "divided by" the calculations for incidence and prevalence can be expressed as follows:

Incidence Rate = Number of New Cases within a Given Time Period / Number of People at Risk of Getting the Disease

Prevalence Rate = Total Number of Cases at a Single Point in Time / Number of People at Risk of Getting the Disease

Multiply the the result by 100 or 1000 to get the number of person to get the number of cases per 100 or 1000, respectively.

Finally, remember that incidence and prevalence statistics are only estimates and a not a perfectly exact reflection of the population being measured. For example, for some health disorders the the incidence rate can be greater than the actual number of people affected by a health condition. A typical example is incidence reports for the common cold. Many individuals may get a common cold two or more times in a given year and therefore will be counted multiple times in incidence statistics even though they are only one person.

Likewise, some prevalence measures estimating the occurrence of a particular cancer type, for instance, may include persons in remission where other prevalence estimates do not. Thus, when reviewing incidence and prevalence reports it is important to not only understand the limitations of each but also the methodology researchers used to report a final estimate.

Sources of Morbidity Statistics

Morbidity statistics are aggregated and collected by a number of organizations. Some organizations that collect this data include:

1. Hospitals and clinics
2. Disease and cancer registries
3. Communicable disease reporting surveillance public health agencies
4. Vital statistics
5. Surveys
6. Health and life insurance plans

Mortality and Disease

One final important indicator of the health status of populations is mortality. Mortality literally means "death" and therefore a mortality rate is the percentage of death in a population in any given time. Importantly, there are a number of mortality rates including, but not limited to, the child mortality rate, infant mortality rate, maternal mortality rate, and age-specific mortality. The crude mortality rate is simply the total number of deaths per 1,000 people, regardless of age, gender, disease, etc. Therefore, the calculation of the crude mortality rate is:

Annual Mortality Rate from All Causes = (Total Number of Deaths in One Year from All Causes / Number of Persons in Population at Mid-Year) x 1,000

Where "/" means "divided by" and "*" means "multiplied by" and the part of formula enclosed in parentheses "( )" is to be performed first.

Sources of Mortality Statistics

The Centers for Disease Control and Prevention (CDC) is the agency that oversees public health in the United States. While the National Institutes of Health is the nation's primary health care research agency, the CDC primary focus is on the health of the population as a whole, and instead of researching disease concentrates instead on the prevention and control of disease outbreaks by primarily studying disease transmission. CDC online resources provide basic information about illness and disease but focus on communicating information about the impact of health conditions on large populations. A vast amount of text and data are available on the CDC website at http://www.cdc.gov/

Most mortality statistics are derived from data from individual death certificates. Primary on death certificates is the identification of the cause of death, frequently abbreviated as COD. Death certificates in the United States generally report two CODs, an **immediate COD** and an **underlying COD**. For example, for leukemia patients a common immediate cause of death is sepsis caused by the underlying cause of death, leukemia.

In the United States, aggregated mortality data and statistics can be found by searching:

1. The **National Death Index (NDI)** from the National Center for Health Statistics http://www.cdc.gov/nchs/ndi.htm

2. The **Morbidity and Mortality Weekly Report** from the Centers for Disease Control and Prevention (CDC) http://www.cdc.gov/mmwr/

3. State vital records. Links to each state agency responsible for that state's vital records can be found at http://www.cdc.gov/nchs/w2w.htm

4. Tumor registries. Links to tumor registries can be found at http://apps.nccd.cdc.gov/dcpc_Programs

Whiplash Journal Articles

Andersen, T. E., Elklit, A., & Brink, O. (2013). PTSD Symptoms Mediate the Effect of Attachment on Pain and Somatisation after Whiplash Injury. *Clinical Practice and Epidemiology in Mental Health: CP & EMH, 9*, 75–83. http://doi.org/10.2174/1745017901309010075

Berglund, A., Alfredsson, L., Jensen, I., Bodin, L., & Nygren, Å. (2003). Occupant- and crash-related factors associated with the risk of whiplash injury. *Annals of Epidemiology, 13*(1), 66–72. http://doi.org/10.1016/S1047-2797(02)00252-1

Berglund, A., Alfredsson, L., Jensen, I., Cassidy, J. D., & Nygren, Å. (2001). The association between exposure to a rear-end collision and future health complaints. *Journal of Clinical Epidemiology, 54*(8), 851–856. http://doi.org/10.1016/S0895-4356(00)00369-3

Berglund, A., Bodin, L., Jensen, I., Wiklund, A., & Alfredsson, L. (2006). The influence of prognostic factors on neck pain intensity, disability, anxiety and depression over a 2-year period in subjects with acute whiplash injury. *Pain, 125*(3), 244–256. http://doi.org/10.1016/j.pain.2006.05.026

Bhatt, Y. M., & de Carpentier, J. P. (2012). Musical hallucination following whiplash injury: case report and literature review. *The Journal of Laryngology and Otology, 126*(6), 615–8. http://doi.org/10.1017/S0022215112000242

Binder, A. (2007). The diagnosis and treatment of nonspecific neck pain and whiplash. *Europa Medicophysica, 43*(1), 79–89.

Buitenhuis, J., de Jong, P. J., Jaspers, J. P. C., & Groothoff, J. W. (2006). Relationship between posttraumatic stress disorder symptoms and the course of whiplash complaints. *Journal of Psychosomatic Research, 61*(5), 681–689. http://doi.org/10.1016/j.jpsychores.2006.07.008

Buitenhuis, J., Spanjer, J., & Fidler, V. (2003). Recovery from acute whiplash: the role of coping styles. *Spine, 28*(9), 896–901. http://doi.org/10.1097/01.BRS.0000058720.56061.2A

Carroll, L. J., Cassidy, J. D., & Côté, P. (2006). The role of pain coping strategies in prognosis after whiplash injury: Passive coping predicts slowed recovery. *Pain, 124*(1-2), 18–26. http://doi.org/10.1016/j.pain.2006.03.012

Carroll, L. J., Holm, L. W., Hogg-Johnson, S., Côté, P., Cassidy, J. D., Haldeman, S., ... Guzman, J. (2008). Course and Prognostic Factors for Neck Pain in Whiplash-Associated Disorders (WAD). *European Spine Journal, 17*(Suppl 1), 83–92. http://doi.org/10.1007/s00586-008-0628-7

Carroll, L. J., Holm, L. W., Hogg-Johnson, S., Côtè, P., Cassidy, J. D., Haldeman, S., ... Guzman, J. (2009). Course and Prognostic Factors for Neck Pain in Whiplash-Associated Disorders (WAD). Results of the Bone and Joint Decade 2000-2010 Task Force on Neck Pain and Its Associated Disorders. *Journal of Manipulative and Physiological Therapeutics, 32*(2 SUPPL.). http://doi.org/10.1016/j.jmpt.2008.11.014

Carroll, L. J., Liu, Y., Holm, L. W., Cassidy, J. D., & Cote, P. (2011). Pain-Related Emotions in Early Stages of Recovery in Whiplash-Associated Disorders: Their Presence, Intensity, and Association With Pain Recovery. *Psychosomatic Medicine.* http://doi.org/10.1097/PSY.0b013e31822f991a

Chen, H., Yang, K. H., & Wang, Z. (2009). Biomechanics of whiplash injury. *Chinese Journal of Traumatology = Zhonghua Chuang Shang Za Zhi / Chinese Medical Association, 12*(5), 305–314. http://doi.org/10.3760/cma.j.issn.1008-1275.2009.05.011

Côté, P., Cassidy, J. D., & Carroll, L. (2003). The epidemiology of neck pain: what we have learned from our population-based studies. *The Journal of the Canadian Chiropractic Association, 47*(4), 284–290.

Côté, P., Hogg-Johnson, S., Cassidy, J. D., Carroll, L., & Frank, J. W. (2001). The association between neck pain intensity, physical functioning, depressive symptomatology and time-to-claim-closure after whiplash. *Journal of Clinical Epidemiology, 54*(3), 275–286. http://doi.org/10.1016/S0895-4356(00)00319-X

Epstein, J. B., & Klasser, G. D. (2011). Whiplash-associated disorders and temporomandibular symptoms following motor-vehicle collisions.

Quintessence International (Berlin, Germany : 1985), *42*(1), e1–e14.

Ferrari, R., Kwan, O., Russell, A. S., Pearce, J. M. S., & Schrader, H. (1999). The best approach to the problem of whiplash? One ticket to Lithuania, please. *Clinical and Experimental Rheumatology*, *17*(3), 321–326.

Ferrari, R., Russell, A. S., & Richter, M. (2001). Epidemiology of whiplash injuries: an international dilemma. *Der Orthopade*, *30*(8), 551–558. http://doi.org/10.1136/ard.58.1.1

Freeman, M. D., Croft, A. C., & Rossignol, A. M. (1998). "Whiplash associated disorders: redefining whiplash and its management" by the Quebec Task Force. A critical evaluation. *Spine*, *23*(9), 1043–1049. http://doi.org/10.1097/00007632-199805010-00015

Freeman, M. D., Croft, A. C., Rossignol, A. M., Centeno, C. J., & Elkins, W. L. (2006a). Chronic neck pain and whiplash: a case-control study of the relationship between acute whiplash injuries and chronic neck pain. *Pain Research & Management : The Journal of the Canadian Pain Society = Journal de La Société Canadienne Pour Le Traitement de La Douleur*, *11*(2), 79–83. Retrieved from http://www.pubmedcentral.nih.gov/articlerender.fcgi?artid=2585479&tool=pmcentrez&rendertype=abstract

Freeman, M. D., Croft, A. C., Rossignol, A. M., Centeno, C. J., & Elkins, W. L. (2006b). Chronic neck pain and whiplash: a case-control study of the relationship between acute whiplash injuries and chronic neck pain. *Pain Research & Management*, *11*(2), 79–83. Retrieved from http://www.pubmedcentral.nih.gov/articlerender.fcgi?artid=2585479&tool=pmcentrez&rendertype=abstract

Gellhorn, A. C. (2011). Cervical Facet-Mediated Pain. *Physical Medicine and Rehabilitation Clinics of North America*. http://doi.org/10.1016/j.pmr.2011.02.006

Giannoudis, P. V, Mehta, S. S., & Tsiridis, E. (2007). Incidence and outcome of whiplash injury after multiple trauma. *Spine (Phila Pa 1976)*, *32*(7), 776–781. http://doi.org/10.1097/01.brs.0000259223.77957.76\r00007632-200704010-00013 [pii]

Häggman-Henrikson, B., List, T., Westergren, H. T., & Axelsson, S. H. (2013). Temporomandibular disorder pain after whiplash trauma: a systematic review. *Journal of Orofacial Pain, 27*(3), 217–26. http://doi.org/10.11607/jop.1027

Harder, S., Veilleux, M., & Suissa, S. (1998). The effect of sociodemographic and crash-related factors on the prognosis of whiplash. *Journal of Clinical Epidemiology, 51*(5), 377–384. http://doi.org/10.1016/S0895-4356(98)00011-0

Hartling, L., Pickett, W., & Brison, R. J. (2002). Derivation of a clinical decision rule for whiplash associated disorders among individuals involved in rear-end collisions. *Accident Analysis and Prevention, 34*(4), 531–539. http://doi.org/10.1016/S0001-4575(01)00051-3

Holm, L. W., Carroll, L. J., Cassidy, J. D., Hogg-Johnson, S., Côté, P., Guzman, J., … Haldeman, S. (2008). The Burden and Determinants of Neck Pain in Whiplash-Associated Disorders After Traffic Collisions. *European Spine Journal, 17*(Suppl 1), 52–59. http://doi.org/10.1007/s00586-008-0625-x

Jaspers, J. P. (1998). Whiplash and post-traumatic stress disorder. *Disabil Rehabil, 20*, 397–404. Retrieved from http://www.ncbi.nlm.nih.gov/entrez/query.fcgi?cmd=Retrieve&db=PubMed&dopt=Citation&list_uids=9846239

Jaspers, J. P. C. (1998a). Whiplash and post-traumatic stress disorder. *Disability & Rehabilitation*.

Jaspers, J. P. C. Whiplash and post-traumatic stress disorder, 20 Disabil Rehabil 397–404 (1998). Retrieved from http://www.ncbi.nlm.nih.gov/entrez/query.fcgi?cmd=Retrieve&db=PubMed&dopt=Citation&list_uids=9846239

Jensen, T. S., Kasch, H., Bach, F. W., Bendix, T., & Kongsted, A. (2010). [Definition, classification and epidemiology of whiplash]. *Ugeskrift for Laeger, 172*(24), 1812–1814. http://doi.org/VP02100049 [pii]

Lind, B. (2001). Frontiers in Whiplash Trauma, Clinical & Biomechanical. *Spine*. http://doi.org/10.1097/00007632-200111150-00028

Lonnberg, F. (2001). [Whiplash. Epidemiology, diagnosis and treatment]. *Ugeskr Laeger*, *163*(16), 2231–2236. Retrieved from http://www.ncbi.nlm.nih.gov/entrez/query.fcgi?cmd=Retrieve&db=PubMed&dopt=Citation&list_uids=11344657

Lønnberg, F. (2001). Whiplash. Epidemiology, diagnosis and treatment. *Ugeskrift for Laeger*, *163*(16), 2231–2236.

Mayou, R., & Radanov, B. P. (1996). Whiplash neck injury. *Journal of Psychosomatic Research*. http://doi.org/10.1016/0022-3999(95)00586-2

Miettinen, T., Lindgren, K. A., Airaksinen, O., & Leino, E. (2002). Whiplash injuries in Finland: A prospective 1-year follow-up study. *Clinical and Experimental Rheumatology*, *20*(3), 399–402.

Montfoort, I., Frens, M. A., Koes, B. W., Lagers-van Haselen, G. C., de Zeeuw, C. I., & Verhagen, A. P. (2008). Tragedy of conducting a clinical trial; generic alert system needed. *Journal of Clinical Epidemiology*, *61*(5), 415–418. http://doi.org/10.1016/j.jclinepi.2007.06.004

Myran, R., Hagen, K., Svebak, S., Nygaard, O., & Zwart, J.-A. (2011). Headache and musculoskeletal complaints among subjects with self reported whiplash injury: the HUNT-2 study. *BMC Musculoskeletal Disorders*, *12*, 129. http://doi.org/10.1186/1471-2474-12-129

Ngo, T., Stupar, M., Côté, P., Boyle, E., & Shearer, H. (2010). A study of the test-retest reliability of the self-perceived general recovery and self-perceived change in neck pain questions in patients with recent whiplash-associated disorders. *European Spine Journal*, *19*(6), 957–962. http://doi.org/10.1007/s00586-010-1289-x

Obermann, M., Nebel, K., Riegel, A., Thiemann, D., Yoon, M. S., Keidel, M., ... Katsarava, Z. (2010). Incidence and predictors of chronic headache attributed to whiplash injury. *Cephalalgia*, *30*(5), 528–534. http://doi.org/10.1111/j.1468-2982.2009.01972.x

Rooker, J., Bannister, M., Amirfeyz, R., Squires, B., Gargan, M., & Bannister, G. (2010). Whiplash injury: 30-year follow-up of a single series. *The Journal of Bone and Joint Surgery. British Volume*, 92(6), 853–855. http://doi.org/10.1302/0301-620X.92B6.23404

Siegmund, G. P., & Brault, J. J. R. (2000). Role of cervical muscles during whiplash. In *Frontiers in whiplash trauma: clinical and biomechanical* (pp. 295–320). Retrieved from http://books.google.com/books?hl=en&lr=&id=Zm1PavZOmaIC&pgis=1

Sjaastad, O., Fredriksen, T. A., Båtnes, J., Petersen, H. C., & Bakketeig, L. S. (2006). Whiplash in individuals with known pre-accident, clinical neck status. *Journal of Headache and Pain*, 7(1), 9–20. http://doi.org/10.1007/s10194-006-0270-x

Stewart, M. J., Maher, C. G., Refshauge, K. M., Herbert, R. D., Bogduk, N., & Nicholas, M. (2007). Randomized controlled trial of exercise for chronic whiplash-associated disorders. *Pain*, 128(1-2), 59–68. http://doi.org/S0304-3959(06)00455-6 [pii] 10.1016/j.pain.2006.08.030

Styrke, J., Stålnacke, B.-M., Bylund, P.-O., Sojka, P., & Björnstig, U. (2012). A 10-year incidence of acute whiplash injuries after road traffic crashes in a defined population in northern Sweden. *PM & R : The Journal of Injury, Function, and Rehabilitation*, 4(10), 739–47. http://doi.org/10.1016/j.pmrj.2012.05.010

Suissa, S. (2003). Risk factors of poor prognosis after whiplash injury. *Pain Research & Management : The Journal of the Canadian Pain Society = Journal de La Société Canadienne Pour Le Traitement de La Douleur*, 8(2), 69–75. Retrieved from http://www.ncbi.nlm.nih.gov/pubmed/12879136

Suissa, S., Harder, S., & Veilleux, M. (2001). The relation between initial symptoms and signs and the prognosis of whiplash. *European Spine Journal*, 10(1), 44–49. http://doi.org/10.1007/s005860000220

Wenzel, H. G., Mykletun, A., & Nilsen, T. I. L. (2009). Symptom profile of persons self-reporting whiplash: A Norwegian population-based study (HUNT 2). *European Spine Journal*, 18(9), 1363–1370.

http://doi.org/10.1007/s00586-009-1106-6

Yadla, S., Ratliff, J. K., & Harrop, J. S. (2008). Whiplash: Diagnosis, treatment, and associated injuries. *Current Reviews in Musculoskeletal Medicine.* http://doi.org/10.1007/s12178-007-9008-x

Yang, X., Côté, P., Cassidy, J. D., & Carroll, L. (2007). Association between body mass index and recovery from whiplash injuries: a cohort study. *American Journal of Epidemiology, 165*(9), 1063–1069. http://doi.org/10.1093/aje/kwk110

Whiplash Internet Articles and Research

BMC Public Health | Full text | The return. (2015). Retrieved on February 2, 2015, from http://www.biomedcentral.com/1471-2458/14/113.

EPIDEMIOLOGY OF WHIPLASH ASSOCIATED DISORDERS. (2015). Retrieved on February 2, 2015, from http://autoinjurieswhiplash.blogspot.com/2013/01/epidemiology-of-whiplash-associated.html.

Epidemiology of whiplash: an international dilemma. (2015). Retrieved on February 2, 2015, from http://ard.bmj.com/content/58/1/1.

Full Text: Whiplash: Social Interventions and Solutions. (2015). Retrieved on February 2, 2015, from https://jrheum.com/subscribers/08/12/2300.html.

Michael D Freeman, MedDr, PhD, MPH | Public Health & Preventive .... (2015). Retrieved on February 2, 2015, from http://www.ohsu.edu/xd/education/schools/school-of-medicine/departments/clinical-departments/public-health/people/michael-d-freeman-phd-mph-d.cfm.

Neck Injury after Whiplash Trauma in a Defined Population in .... (2015). Retrieved on February 2, 2015, from http://omicsonline.org/epidemiology-open-access-abstract.php?abstract_id=30765.

Online CE Courses | Whiplash. (2015). Retrieved on February 2, 2015, from https://www.milestonece.com/course-info/online-ce-courses-%7C-whiplash.

The Epidemiology of Neck Pain. (2015). Retrieved on February 2, 2015, from http://www.digital-doc.com/neckpain.htm.

Whiplash (medicine). (2015). Retrieved on February 2, 2015, from http://en.wikipedia.org/wiki/Whiplash_(medicine).

Whiplash and Cervical Spine Injury | Patient.co.uk. (2015). Retrieved on February 2, 2015, from http://www.patient.co.uk/doctor/whiplash-and-cervical-spine-injury.

Whiplash. (2015). Retrieved on February 2, 2015, from http://www.srisd.com/consumer_site/epidemiology.htm.

Widespread Pain Following Whiplash. (2015). Retrieved on February 2, 2015, from https://jrheum.com/abstracts/abstracts06/13/1210.html.

Chiropractic Resource Organization. (2015). *25 Years of Whiplash Research*. Retrieved on February 2, 2015, from http://www.chiro.org/LINKS/ABSTRACTS/25_Years_of_Whiplash_Researc

CHAPTER 4
RISK FACTORS
&
CAUSES

During the course of researching health conditions many people use the the concepts of risk factors and causes interchangeably. However, it is important to remember in medicine these concepts have unique meanings. This Chapter will define these commonly confused concepts and explain the risk factors and causes of Whiplash.

Risk Factors for Disease

A risk factor is any aspect or circumstance in a person's life that predisposes or makes it more likely that the person will acquire a particular health condition. Essentially, risk factors are anything that increases the chance of developing a disease. Some examples of risk factors for many diseases include age, a family history of certain conditions, use of tobacco products, being exposed to radiation or certain chemicals, infection with certain viruses or bacteria, and certain genetic makeups.

If you discover you have a risk factor for a certain condition it doesn't necessarily mean that you will get that disease. It only means your chances of the getting the disease are higher when compared to other individuals similar to yourself who are not exposed to the stated risk factor(s). In this regard, it is important to note that risk factors and causes are essentially measures of **correlation** or **causation**. The distinction between correlation and causation is very important in medical research.

Correlation means two factors are related and also expresses in statistical terms how closely the two factors are related. For example, there exists a correlation between age and food allergies, as children are about twice as likely as adults of having food allergies. However, this doesn't mean that being a child *causes* food allergies.

Causes of Disease

This leads us to the definition of causation and the dual nature of cause and effect. In medicine causation essentially implies change in the normal constitution or functioning of the body as the result of the introduction of a second factor (the cause). To return to the the previous example, food allergies are most commonly due to an allergen-antibody interaction, therefore the cause can be said to be the allergen-antibody interaction and the effect (or manifestation of the cause) is the food allergy (and not being a child). Researchers have discovered the reason that children are more likely to have food allergies is because their immune systems are not as well-developed as adults and their bodies are more likely to mistakenly identify certain foods as "harmful" and trigger the allergen-antibody reaction.

Similarly, when studying risk factors, another important terminology distinction is between **effect** and **association**. Both effect and association are quantitative measures of the increased or decreased prevalence, rate, or risk for disease in an exposed population but epidemiologists use the term effect when the risk factor can be changed and association when it cannot be changed. For example, one effect of obesity may be uterine cancer but this risk factor can be reduced or eliminated by losing weight. On the other hand, uterine cancer is only associated with women, but even though a hysterectomy will remove the uterus the patient will still remain a woman.

Most research you come across will clearly distinguish between correlation/causation and effect/association. Further, as you will soon discover, nearly all advances in research into illness and disease first establish correlation or association but only later establish causation or effect. For example, through observation researchers were able to quickly ascertain that smokers were more likely to develop lung cancer, meaning that there exists a correlation between smoking and lung cancer and was higher than between non-smoking and lung cancer. However, further research was needed to determine that smoking, and not some other attribute common among smokers, was a cause of lung cancer.

An extreme, and intuitively far-fetched but common example to illustrate our point is the story of Inept Researcher A. Among office workers, Inept

Researcher A notices that workers who take many rest breaks have more sick days due to respiratory illness than workers who take fewer breaks. Inept Researcher A quickly concludes that "work breaks cause respiratory disease" and in his haste forgoes peer-reviewed journals and publishes his "landmark discovery" on his own, including a recommendation that government move quickly to establish laws prohibiting all work rest breaks. Soon, however, All-Star Researcher B reads the article and does her own analysis of the data. In no time at all, All-Star Researcher B is able to debunk Inept Researcher A's conclusions by correctly determining that work breaks do not cause respiratory illness. She further hypothesizes (and is later proven correct) it is not the break itself causing respiratory illness; but what people do on these work breaks, namely smoking cigarettes that is the real cause of respiratory illness in persons taking frequent work breaks.

While Inept Researcher A's "discovery" may seem intuitively false, it is not always this easy to correctly identify incorrect or illogical conclusions of cause and effect. Therefore, during the course of your research take special note to distinguish statements of correlation with assertions of cause and effect or be prepared to suffer consequences of falsely jumping to erroneous conclusions.

Whiplash Journal Articles

Awerbuch, M. S. (1992). Whiplash in Australia: Illness or injury? *Medical Journal of Australia*.

Banic, B., Petersen-Felix, S., Andersen, O. K., Radanov, B. P., Villiger, P. M., Arendt-Nielsen, L., & Curatolo, M. (2004). Evidence for spinal cord hypersensitivity in chronic pain after whiplash injury and in fibromyalgia. *Pain*, *107*(1-2), 7–15. http://doi.org/10.1016/j.pain.2003.05.001

Barak, S. (2013). [The relationship between whiplash injury and temporomandibular joint dysfunction]. *Harefuah*, *152*(10), 612–4, 622. Retrieved from http://www.ncbi.nlm.nih.gov/pubmed/24450037

Binder, A. (2007). The diagnosis and treatment of nonspecific neck pain and whiplash. *Europa Medicophysica*, *43*(1), 79–89.

Bodack, M. P., Tunkel, R. S., Marini, S. G., & Nagler, W. (1998a). Spinal accessory nerve palsy as a cause of pain after whiplash injury: case report. *J Pain Symptom Manage*, *15*(5), 321–328. http://doi.org/S0885-3924(98)00008-6 [pii]

Bodack, M. P., Tunkel, R. S., Marini, S. G., & Nagler, W. Spinal accessory nerve palsy as a cause of pain after whiplash injury: case report., 15 Journal of pain and symptom management 321–328 (1998). http://doi.org/10.1016/S0885-3924(98)00008-6

Castro, W. H. M., Meyer, S. J., Becke, M. E. R., Nentwig, C. G., Hein, M. F., Ercan, B. I., ... Du Chesne, A. E. (2001). No stress - No whiplash? Prevalence of "whiplash" symptoms following exposure to a placebo rear-end collision. *International Journal of Legal Medicine*, *114*(6), 316–322. http://doi.org/10.1007/s004140000193

Cavanaugh, J. M., Lu, Y., Chen, C., & Kallakuri, S. (2006). Pain generation in lumbar and cervical facet joints. *The Journal of Bone and Joint Surgery. American Volume*, *88 Suppl 2*, 63–67. http://doi.org/10.2106/JBJS.E.01411

Chen, H., Yang, K. H., & Wang, Z. (2009). Biomechanics of whiplash injury.

Chinese Journal of Traumatology = Zhonghua Chuang Shang Za Zhi / Chinese Medical Association, 12(5), 305–314. http://doi.org/10.3760/cma.j.issn.1008-1275.2009.05.011

Colicchia, G., Zollman, D., Wiesner, H., & Sen, A. I. (2008). Kinematics of a Head-Neck Model Simulating Whiplash. *The Physics Teacher*. http://doi.org/10.1119/1.2834528

Curatolo, M., Petersen-Felix, S., Arendt-Nielsen, L., Giani, C., Zbinden, A. M., & Radanov, B. P. (2001). Central hypersensitivity in chronic pain after whiplash injury. *The Clinical Journal of Pain, 17*(4), 306–315. http://doi.org/10.1097/00002508-200112000-00004

Davis, C. G. (2013). Mechanisms of chronic pain from whiplash injury. *Journal of Forensic and Legal Medicine*. http://doi.org/10.1016/j.jflm.2012.05.004

Dispenza, F., De Stefano, A., Mathur, N., Croce, A., & Gallina, S. (2010). Benign paroxysmal positional vertigo following whiplash injury: a myth or a reality? *American Journal of Otolaryngology, 32*(5), 376–80. http://doi.org/10.1016/j.amjoto.2010.07.009

Dispenza, F., De Stefano, A., Mathur, N., Croce, A., & Gallina, S. (2011). Benign paroxysmal positional vertigo following whiplash injury: a myth or a reality? *Am J Otolaryngol, 32*(5), 376–80. http://doi.org/10.1016/j.amjoto.2010.07.009

Duffy, M. F., Stuberg, W., DeJong, S., Gold, K. V, & Nystrom, N. A. Case report: whiplash-associated disorder from a low-velocity bumper car collision: history, evaluation, and surgery., 29 Spine 1881–1884 (2004). http://doi.org/10.1097/01.brs.0000137064.85554.fa

Endo, K., Ichimaru, K., Komagata, M., & Yamamoto, K. (2006). Cervical vertigo and dizziness after whiplash injury. *European Spine Journal, 15*(6), 886–890. http://doi.org/10.1007/s00586-005-0970-y

Ferrari, R. (2002). Prevention of chronic pain after whiplash. *Emergency Medicine Journal : EMJ, 19*(6), 526–530.

http://doi.org/10.1136/emj.19.6.526

Ferrari, R. (2006). Auditory symptoms in whiplash patients - could earwax occlusion be a benign cause? *Australian Family Physician.*, *35*(5), 367–368.

Freeman, M. D., Croft, A. C., Rossignol, A. M., Centeno, C. J., & Elkins, W. L. (2006a). Chronic neck pain and whiplash: a case-control study of the relationship between acute whiplash injuries and chronic neck pain. *Pain Res Manag.*, *11*(2), 79–83.

Freeman, M. D., Croft, A. C., Rossignol, A. M., Centeno, C. J., & Elkins, W. L. (2006b). Chronic neck pain and whiplash: a case-control study of the relationship between acute whiplash injuries and chronic neck pain. *Pain Research & Management : The Journal of the Canadian Pain Society = Journal de La Société Canadienne Pour Le Traitement de La Douleur*, *11*(2), 79–83. Retrieved from http://www.pubmedcentral.nih.gov/articlerender.fcgi?artid=2585479&tool=pmcentrez&rendertype=abstract

Freeman, M. D., Croft, A. C., Rossignol, A. M., Weaver, D. S., & Reiser, M. (1999). A review and methodologic critique of the literature refuting whiplash syndrome. *Spine*, *24*(1), 86–96. http://doi.org/10.1097/00007632-199901010-00023

Giannoudis, P. V, Mehta, S. S., & Tsiridis, E. (2007). Incidence and outcome of whiplash injury after multiple trauma. *Spine (Phila Pa 1976)*, *32*(7), 776–781. http://doi.org/10.1097/01.brs.0000259223.77957.76\r00007632-200704010-00013 [pii]

Giannoudis, P. V, Mehta, S. S., & Tsiridis, E. (2007). Incidence and outcome of whiplash injury after multiple trauma. *Spine*, *32*(7), 776–781. http://doi.org/10.1097/01.brs.0000259223.77957.76

Gimse, R., Tjell, C., Bjørgen, I. A., & Saunte, C. (1996). Disturbed eye movements after whiplash due to injuries to the posture control system. *Journal of Clinical and Experimental Neuropsychology*, *18*(2), 178–186. http://doi.org/10.1080/01688639608408273

Gosselin, G., Rassoulian, H., & Brown, I. (2004). Effects of neck extensor muscles fatigue on balance. *Clinical Biomechanics, 19*(5), 473–479. http://doi.org/10.1016/j.clinbiomech.2004.02.001

Haas, D. C. Traumatic-event headaches., 4 BMC neurology 17 (2004). http://doi.org/10.1186/1471-2377-4-17

Krakenes, J., Kaale, B. R., Moen, G., Nordli, H., Gilhus, N. E., & Rorvik, J. (2002). MRI assessment of the alar ligaments in the late stage of whiplash injury - A study of structural abnormalities and observer agreement. *Neuroradiology, 44*(7), 617–624. http://doi.org/10.1007/s00234-002-0799-6

Lo, Y.-L., Tan, Y.-E., Fook-Chong, S., Boolsambatra, P., Yue, W.-M., Chan, L.-L., & Tan, S.-B. (2007). Role of spinal inhibitory mechanisms in whiplash injuries. *Journal of Neurotrauma, 24*(6), 1055–1067. http://doi.org/10.1089/neu.2006.0222

Malanga, G., & Peter, J. (2005a). Whiplash injuries. *Current Pain and Headache Reports, 9*(5), 322–325. http://doi.org/10.1007/s11916-005-0007-6

Malanga, G., & Peter, J. (2005b). Whiplash injuries. *Curr Pain and Headache Rep, 9*(5), 322–5. Retrieved from http://www.ncbi.nlm.nih.gov/pubmed/16157060

Mealy, K., Brennan, H., & Fenelon, G. C. (1986). *Early mobilization of acute whiplash injuries. British medical journal (Clinical research ed.)* (Vol. 292).

Nacci, a, Ferrazzi, M., Berrettini, S., Panicucci, E., Matteucci, J., Bruschini, L., … Fattori, B. (2011). Vestibular and stabilometric findings in whiplash injury and minor head trauma. *Acta Otorhinolaryngologica Italica : Organo Ufficiale Della Società Italiana Di Otorinolaringologia E Chirurgia Cervico-Facciale, 31*(6), 378–89. Retrieved from http://www.pubmedcentral.nih.gov/articlerender.fcgi?artid=3272873&tool=pmcentrez&rendertype=abstract

Nederhand, M. J., Hermens, H. J., IJzerman, M. J., Turk, D. C., & Zilvold, G. (2002). Cervical muscle dysfunction in chronic whiplash-associated disorder grade 2: the relevance of the trauma. *Spine, 27*(10), 1056–1061. http://doi.org/10.1097/00007632-200205150-00010

Nurata, H., Yilmaz, M. B., Borcek, A. O., Oner, A. Y., & Baykaner, M. K. (2012). Retropharyngeal hematoma secondary to whiplash injury in childhood: A case report. *Turkish Neurosurgery*, *22*(4), 521–523. http://doi.org/10.5137/1019-5149.JTN.4011-10.0

O'Neill, B. (2000). Head restraints - The neglected countermeasure. *Accident Analysis and Prevention*, *32*(2), 143–150. http://doi.org/10.1016/S0001-4575(99)00057-3

Padberg, M., De Bruijn, S. F. T. M., & Tavy, D. L. J. (2007). Neck pain in chronic whiplash syndrome treated with botulinum toxin. A double-blind, placebo-controlled clinical trial. *Journal of Neurology*, *254*(3), 290–295. http://doi.org/10.1007/s00415-006-0317-6

Panjabi, M. M., Cholewicki, J., Nibu, K., Babat, L. B., & Dvorak, J. (1998). Simulation of whiplash trauma using whole cervical spine specimens. *Spine*, *23*(1), 17–24. http://doi.org/10.1097/00007632-199801010-00005

Pinfold, M., Niere, K. R., O'Leary, E. F., Hoving, J. L., Green, S., & Buchbinder, R. (2004). Validity and internal consistency of a whiplash-specific disability measure. *Spine*, *29*(3), 263–268. http://doi.org/10.1097/01.BRS.0000107238.15526.4C

Schofferman, J., Bogduk, N., & Slosar, P. Chronic whiplash and whiplash-associated disorders: an evidence-based approach., 15 The Journal of the American Academy of Orthopaedic Surgeons 596–606 (2007). http://doi.org/15/10/596 [pii]

Schrader, H., Stovner, L. J., & Eisenmenger, W. (2012). Doubtful nosological validity of the chronic whiplash syndrome. *Der Orthopäde*. http://doi.org/10.1007/s00132-011-1868-5

Stålnacke, B. M. (2009). Relationship between symptoms and psychological factors five years after whiplash injury. *Journal of Rehabilitation Medicine*, *41*(5), 353–359. http://doi.org/10.2340/16501977-0349

Sterner, Y., & Gerdle, B. (2004a). Acute and chronic whiplash disorders - A review. *Journal of Rehabilitation Medicine*.

http://doi.org/10.1080/16501970410030742

Sterner, Y., & Gerdle, B. (2004b). Acute and chronic whiplash disorders--a review. *Journal of Rehabilitation Medicine : Official Journal of the UEMS European Board of Physical and Rehabilitation Medicine*, 36(5), 193–209; quiz 210. http://doi.org/10.1080/16501970410030742

Svensson, M. Y., Aldman, B., Hansson, H. a, Lövsund, P., Seeman, T., Suneson, a, & Örtengren, T. (1993). Pressure Effects in the Spinal Canal during Whiplash Extension Motion: A Possible Cause of Injury to the Cervical Spinal Ganglia. *International IRCOBI Conference on the Biomechanics of Impacts*, (1986), 189–200.

Teasell, R. W. (1998). Whiplash injuries: An update. *Pain Research and Management*, 3(2), 81–90.

Tough, E. A., White, A. R., Richards, S. H., & Campbell, J. L. (2010). *Myofascial trigger point needling for whiplash associated pain--a feasibility study*. Manual therapy (Vol. 15).

Treleaven, J., Jull, G., & Sterling, M. (2003). Dizziness and unsteadiness following whiplash injury: Characteristic features and relationship with cervical joint position error. *Journal of Rehabilitation Medicine*, 35(1), 36–43. http://doi.org/10.1080/16501970306109

Verhagen, A. P., Lewis, M., Schellingerhout, J. M., Heymans, M. W., Dziedzic, K., de Vet, H. C. W., & Koes, B. W. (2011). Do whiplash patients differ from other patients with non-specific neck pain regarding pain, function or prognosis? *Manual Therapy*, 16(5), 456–462. http://doi.org/10.1016/j.math.2011.02.009

Yadla, S., Ratliff, J. K., & Harrop, J. S. (2008). Whiplash: Diagnosis, treatment, and associated injuries. *Current Reviews in Musculoskeletal Medicine*. http://doi.org/10.1007/s12178-007-9008-x

Yu, L. J., Stokell, R., & Treleaven, J. (2011). The effect of neck torsion on postural stability in subjects with persistent whiplash. *Manual Therapy*, 16(4), 339–343. http://doi.org/10.1016/j.math.2010.12.006

Whiplash Internet Articles and Research

Automobile Car Accident Information and Symptoms, Austin .... (2015). Retrieved on February 2, 2015, from http://www.kapsner.com/automobile_car_accident_pain.asp.

Cervical Sprain and Strain. (2015). Retrieved on February 2, 2015, from http://emedicine.medscape.com/article/306176-overview.

Factors Affecting the Whiplash Injury. (2015). Retrieved on February 2, 2015, from http://www.spine-health.com/conditions/neck-pain/factors-affecting-whiplash-injury.

Hearing Matters: In Whiplash Injury, Audiological Symptoms... : The .... (2015). Retrieved on February 2, 2015, from http://journals.lww.com/thehearingjournal/Fulltext/2013/02000/Hearing_Matt

Most common injuries after a car accident in California | Severe .... (2015). Retrieved on February 2, 2015, from http://www.severeaccidents.com/california-auto/most-common-injuries-after-a-car-accident-in-california/.

Occipital Neuralgia. (2015). Retrieved on February 2, 2015, from http://www.healthgrades.com/conditions/occipital-neuralgia.

Risks and Symptoms of Graves' Disease & Hyperthyroidism. (2015). Retrieved on February 2, 2015, from http://thyroid.about.com/od/hyperthyroidismgraves/a/risks-symptoms.htm.

The risk of whiplash. (2015). Retrieved on February 2, 2015, from http://www.sciencedirect.com/science/article/pii/S0386111213000113.

Vertigo & Dizziness Causes & Risk Factors. (2015). Retrieved on February 2, 2015, from http://www.sharecare.com/health/vertigo-dizziness-causes-risk-factors.

Whiplash Animation. (2015). Retrieved on February 2, 2015, from http://www.spineuniverse.com/conditions/whiplash/whiplash-animation.

Whiplash Injury Lawyers | Patterson Legal Group. (2015). Retrieved on February 2, 2015, from http://pattersonlegalgroup.com/injuries/whiplash-injury-lawyer/.

Whiplash Overview, Causes, Symptoms. (2015). Retrieved on February 2, 2015, from http://www.healthcommunities.com/whiplash/causes-symptoms-of-whiplash.shtml.

Whiplash and Cervical Spine Injury | Patient.co.uk. (2015). Retrieved on February 2, 2015, from http://www.patient.co.uk/doctor/whiplash-and-cervical-spine-injury.

Whiplash and jaw pain: A multifactorial non. (2015). Retrieved on February 2, 2015, from http://www.bcmj.org/article/whiplash-and-jaw-pain-multifactorial-non-structural-relationship.

Whiplash | eOrthopod.com. (2015). Retrieved on February 2, 2015, from http://www.eorthopod.com/whiplash/topic/191.

Whiplash: Predicting Long. (2015). Retrieved on February 2, 2015, from http://www.webmd.com/brain/news/20010625/whiplash-predicting-long-term-problems.

Why Whiplash Matters. (2015). Retrieved on February 2, 2015, from http://www.whiplashprevention.org/Employers/WhiplashMatters/Pages/Defau

whiplash. (2015). Retrieved on February 2, 2015, from http://medical-dictionary.thefreedictionary.com/whiplash.

Chiropractic Resource Organization. (2015). *Whiplash and Neck Injury Information Page.* Retrieved on February 2, 2015, from http://www.chiro.org/LINKS/FULL/Neck_Injury_Q_A.shtml.

Dolinis. (2015). *Risk factors for 'whiplash' in drivers: a cohort study of rear.* Retrieved on February 2, 2015, from http://www.ncbi.nlm.nih.gov/pubmed/9274732.

IHS - International Headache Society. (2015). *HEADACHE ATTRIBUTED*

TO HEAD AND/OR NECK TRAUMA. Retrieved on February 2, 2015, from http://ihs-classification.org/en/02_klassifikation/03_teil2/05.00.00_necktrauma.html.

CHAPTER 5
SYMPTOMS
&
SIGNS

Distinguishing Symtoms from Signs

According to the National Institutes of Health, a symptom is a "physical or mental problem that a person experiences that may indicate a disease or condition." While a sign can mean the same thing noteworthy to the definition of symptom is that symptoms are typically *not* seen **(observed)** by other people and generally can *not* be independently identified **(for diagnosis)** by doctors using medical tests. Signs, on the other hand, can be both **observed** and used to independently **diagnosis** a condition without patient input. Therefore, while the presence or absence of a symptom can not conclusively be used to determine the presence or absence of disease, a sign can be, or cynically speaking, a patient can claim nonexistent symptoms that can not be refuted by doctors but signs can be identified and measured independent of patient input. Common symptoms for many health conditions include fatigue, pain, nausea, and headache. On the other hand, signs of disease often include skin rashes, sweating, uncontrollable bleeding, and difficulties with speech. Notwithstanding "provability," both the accurate portrayl of symptoms and observable signs are critical in disease diagnosis, treatment, and management.

Types of Symptoms

Symptoms of disease can be characterized in a number of ways. First, they can be described by their presence or absence. In this regard, symptoms may be persistent or long-lasting **(chronic)**, ebb and flow at regular or irregular intervals **(relapsing)**, or disappear completely even though the underlying disease may still be present **(remitting)**. Further, some diseases may be **asymptomatic** meaning the underlying disease condition presents no symptoms whatsoever. Frequently, conditions like diabetes and high blood pressure are asymptomatic in that they can be present with no symptoms.

Symptoms can also be classified by the way they impact the "total person." In describing mental disorders in particular, symptoms can be described as **positive** or **negative**. Many people mistakenly imply positive and negative symptoms to mean good and bad symptoms. Instead, positive and negative symptoms should be considered in a more mathematical plus or minus sense. Thus, positive symptoms are feelings (stimulus) in addition to or added to a person's normal spectrum of feelings/stimulus and negative symptoms are feelings/stimulus taken away from the normal spectrum. Therefore, for a mental health disorder like schizophrenia a positive symptom may include hallucinations where a person sees things in addition to things actually present. Conversely, a negative symptom may include a "flat affect" where facial expressions and typical speaking rhythms and changes in tone found in a normal person are absent in a person with Whiplash. Other negative symptoms commonly found in patients with mental health illnesses include taking *less* pleasure in life, speaking *less*, or engaging in *fewer* activities all when compared to persons without mental illness.

Whiplash Journal Articles

Andersen, T. E., Elklit, A., & Brink, O. (2013). PTSD Symptoms Mediate the Effect of Attachment on Pain and Somatisation after Whiplash Injury. *Clinical Practice and Epidemiology in Mental Health: CP & EMH, 9,* 75–83. http://doi.org/10.2174/1745017901309010075

Borenstein, P., Rosenfeld, M., & Gunnarsson, R. (2010). Cognitive symptoms, cervical range of motion and pain as prognostic factors after whiplash trauma. *Acta Neurologica Scandinavica, 122*(4), 278–285. http://doi.org/10.1111/j.1600-0404.2009.01305.x

Buitenhuis, J., de Jong, P. J., Jaspers, J. P. C., & Groothoff, J. W. (2006). Relationship between posttraumatic stress disorder symptoms and the course of whiplash complaints. *Journal of Psychosomatic Research, 61*(5), 681–689. http://doi.org/10.1016/j.jpsychores.2006.07.008

Castro, W. H. M., Meyer, S. J., Becke, M. E. R., Nentwig, C. G., Hein, M. F., Ercan, B. I., ... Du Chesne, A. E. (2001). No stress - No whiplash? Prevalence of "whiplash" symptoms following exposure to a placebo rear-end collision. *International Journal of Legal Medicine, 114*(6), 316–322. http://doi.org/10.1007/s004140000193

Crutebo, S., Nilsson, C., Skillgate, E., & Holm, L. W. (2010). The course of symptoms for whiplash-associated disorders in Sweden: 6-month followup study. *Journal of Rheumatology, 37*(7), 1527–1533. http://doi.org/10.3899/jrheum.091321

Curtis, P., Spanos, A., & Reid, A. (1995). Persistent symptoms after whiplash injuries implications for prognosis and management. *Journal of Clinical Rheumatology : Practical Reports on Rheumatic & Musculoskeletal Diseases, 1*(3), 149–157. http://doi.org/10.1097/00124743-199506000-00004

Daenen, L., Nijs, J., Roussel, N., Wouters, K., Van loo, M., & Cras, P. (2012). Sensorimotor incongruence exacerbates symptoms in patients with chronic whiplash associated disorders: An experimental study. *Rheumatology (United Kingdom), 51*(8), 1492–1499. http://doi.org/10.1093/rheumatology/kes050

Elliott, J. M., Noteboom, J. T., Flynn, T. W., & Sterling, M. (2009). Characterization of acute and chronic whiplash-associated disorders. *The Journal of Orthopaedic and Sports Physical Therapy*, *39*(5), 312–323. http://doi.org/10.2519/jospt.2009.2826

Epstein, J. B., & Klasser, G. D. (2011). Whiplash-associated disorders and temporomandibular symptoms following motor-vehicle collisions. *Quintessence International (Berlin, Germany : 1985)*, *42*(1), e1–e14.

Ettlin, T., Kischka, U., & Kaeser, H. E. Cognitive and psychological disorders following whiplash injury: 2 case reports concerning the controversy between the organic versus the psychogenic etiology of symptoms, 78 Schweizerische Rundschau fur Medizin Praxis = Revue suisse de medecine Praxis 967–969 (1989).

Ettlin, T. M., Kischka, U., Reichmann, S., Radii, E. W., Heim, S., Wengen, D., & Benson, D. F. (1992). Cerebral symptoms after whiplash injury of the neck: a prospective clinical and neuropsychological study of whiplash injury. *Journal of Neurology, Neurosurgery, and Psychiatry*, *55*(10), 943–948. http://doi.org/10.1136/jnnp.55.10.943

Ferrari, R. (2006). Auditory symptoms in whiplash patients - could earwax occlusion be a benign cause? *Australian Family Physician.*, *35*(5), 367–368.

Freeman, M. D., & Croft, A. C. (1998). The controversy over late whiplash: Are chronic symptoms after whiplash real ? In *Whiplash injuries: Current concepts in prevention, diagnosis, and treatment of the cervical whiplash sndrome* (pp. 161–165).

Haldorsen, T., Waterloo, K., Dahl, A., Mellgren, S. I., Davidsen, P. E., & Molin, P. K. (2003). Symptoms and cognitive dysfunction in patients with the late whiplash syndrome. *Applied Neuropsychology*, *10*(3), 170–175. http://doi.org/10.1207/S15324826AN1003_06

Haneline, M. T. (2009). The notion of a "whiplash culture": a review of the evidence. *Journal of Chiropractic Medicine*. http://doi.org/10.1016/j.jcm.2009.04.001

Heise, A. P., Laskin, D. M., & Gervin, A. S. (1992). Incidence of temporomandibular joint symptoms following whiplash injury. *Journal of Oral and Maxillofacial Surgery : Official Journal of the American Association of Oral and Maxillofacial Surgeons, 50*(8), 825–828. http://doi.org/10.1016/0278-2391(92)90273-3

Ide, M., Ide, J., Yamaga, M., & Takagi, K. (2001). Symptoms and signs of irritation of the brachial plexus in whiplash injuries. *The Journal of Bone and Joint Surgery. British Volume, 83*(2), 226–229.

Johansson, M. P., Baann Liane, M. S., Bendix, T., Kasch, H., & Kongsted, A. (2011). Does cervical kyphosis relate to symptoms following whiplash injury? *Manual Therapy, 16*(4), 378–383. http://doi.org/10.1016/j.math.2011.01.004

John, M. T. (2011). Whiplash is likely to be associated with temporomandibular disorder symptoms, but the magnitude of this association is not known. *Journal of Evidence-Based Dental Practice*. http://doi.org/10.1016/j.jebdp.2011.06.013

Jones, A., & Elklit, A. S. K. (2007). The association between gender, coping style and whiplash related symptoms in sufferers of whiplash associated disorder. *Scandinavian Journal of Psychology, 48*(1), 75–80. http://doi.org/10.1111/j.1467-9450.2006.00543.x

Kischka, U., Ettlin, T., Heim, S., & Schmid, G. (1991). Cerebral symptoms following whiplash injury. *European Neurology, 31*(3), 136–140. http://doi.org/10.1159/000116663

Klobas, L., Tegelberg, A., & Axelsson, S. (2004). Symptoms and signs of temporomandibular disorders in individuals with chronic whiplash-associated disorders. *Swed Dent J, 28*(1), 29–36. Retrieved from http://www.ncbi.nlm.nih.gov/entrez/query.fcgi?cmd=Retrieve&db=PubMed&dopt=Citation&list_uids=15129603

Kongsted, A., Sorensen, J. S., Andersen, H., Keseler, B., Jensen, T. S., & Bendix, T. (2008). Are early MRI findings correlated with long-lasting symptoms following whiplash injury? A prospective trial with 1-year follow-up. *European Spine Journal*, *17*(8), 996–1005. http://doi.org/10.1007/s00586-008-0687-9

Krafft, M., Kullgren, A., Sigrun, M., & Ydenius, A. (2005). Influence of crash severity on various whiplash injury symptoms: A study based on real-life rear-end crashes with recorded crash pulses. *Proceedings 19th ESV...*, 1–8. Retrieved from http://www-nrd.nhtsa.dot.gov/pdf/esv/esv19/05-0363-O.pdf

Landrock, C. K., & Souvestre, P. A. (2006). Whiplash-associated disorders and patient traumatic history: a correlation between traumas, symptoms and MVAs. *Journal of Whiplash & Related Disorders*, *5*(2), 25–35. http://doi.org/10.1300/J180v05n02

Linnman, C., Appel, L., Söderlund, A., Frans, Ö., Engler, H., Furmark, T., ... Fredrikson, M. (2009). Chronic whiplash symptoms are related to altered regional cerebral blood flow in the resting state. *European Journal of Pain*, *13*(1), 65–70. http://doi.org/10.1016/j.ejpain.2008.03.001

Magnússon, T. (1994). Extracervical symptoms after whiplash trauma. *Cephalalgia : An International Journal of Headache*, *14*(3), 223–227; discussion 181–182. http://doi.org/10.1046/j.1468-2982.1994.014003223.x

Merrick, D., & Stålnacke, B.-M. (2010). Five years post whiplash injury: Symptoms and psychological factors in recovered versus non-recovered. *BMC Research Notes*, *3*, 190. http://doi.org/10.1186/1756-0500-3-190

Myrtveit, S. M., Skogen, J. C., & Mykletun, A. (2010). P02-315 - Somatic symptoms amongst individuals also reporting whiplash: a Norwegian population-based study (HUSK). *European Psychiatry*. http://doi.org/10.1016/S0924-9338(10)71014-2

Myrtveit, S., Skogen, J., Wenzel, H., & Mykletun, A. (2012). Somatic symptoms beyond those generally associated with a whiplash injury are increased in self-reported chronic whiplash. A population-based cross sectional study: the Hordaland Health Study (HUSK). *BMC Psychiatry*. http://doi.org/10.1186/1471-244X-12-129

Olsnes, B. T. (1989). Neurobehavioral findings in whiplash patients with long-lasting symptoms. *Acta Neurologica Scandinavica, 80*(6), 584–588.

Pedler, A., & Sterling, M. (2013). Patients with chronic whiplash can be subgrouped on the basis of symptoms of sensory hypersensitivity and posttraumatic stress. *Pain, 154*(9), 1640–1648. http://doi.org/10.1016/j.pain.2013.05.005

Pettersson, K., Kärrholm, J., Toolanen, G., & Hildingsson, C. (1995). Decreased width of the spinal canal in patients with chronic symptoms after whiplash injury. *Spine, 20*(15), 1664–1667. http://doi.org/10.1097/00007632-199508000-00003

Radanov, B. P., Mannion, A. F., & Ballinari, P. (2011). Are symptoms of late whiplash specific? A comparison of SCL-90-R symptom profiles of patients with late whiplash and patients with chronic pain due to other types of trauma. *Journal of Rheumatology, 38*(6), 1086–1094. http://doi.org/10.3899/jrheum.101112

Rowlands, R. G., Campbell, I. K., & Kenyon, G. S. (2009). Otological and vestibular symptoms in patients with low grade (Quebec grades one and two) whiplash injury. *The Journal of Laryngology and Otology, 123*(2), 182–185. http://doi.org/10.1017/S0022215108002569

Severinsson, Y., Bunketorp, O., & Wenneberg, B. (2010). Jaw symptoms and signs and the connection to cranial cervical symptoms and post-traumatic stress during the first year after a whiplash trauma. *Disability and Rehabilitation, 32*(24), 1987–1998. http://doi.org/10.3109/09638281003797323

Sjöström, H., Allum, J. H. J., Carpenter, M. G., Adkin, A. L., Honegger, F., & Ettlin, T. (2003). *Trunk sway measures of postural stability during clinical balance tests in patients with chronic whiplash injury symptoms. Spine* (Vol. 28).

Stålnacke, B. M. (2009). Relationship between symptoms and psychological factors five years after whiplash injury. *Journal of Rehabilitation Medicine, 41*(5), 353–359. http://doi.org/10.2340/16501977-0349

Sterling, M., & Chadwick, B. J. (2010). Psychologic processes in daily life with chronic whiplash: relations of posttraumatic stress symptoms and fear-of-pain to hourly pain and uptime. *The Clinical Journal of Pain, 26*(7), 573–582. http://doi.org/10.1097/AJP.0b013e3181e5c25e

Sturzenegger, M., DiStefano, G., Radanov, B. P., & Schnidrig, A. (1994). Presenting symptoms and signs after whiplash injury: the influence of accident mechanisms. *Neurology, 44*(4), 688–693. http://doi.org/10.1212/WNL.44.4.688

Suissa, S., Harder, S., & Veilleux, M. (2001). The relation between initial symptoms and signs and the prognosis of whiplash. *European Spine Journal, 10*(1), 44–49. http://doi.org/10.1007/s005860000220

Sullivan, M. J. L., Thibault, P., Simmonds, M. J., Milioto, M., Cantin, A. P., & Velly, A. M. (2009). Pain, perceived injustice and the persistence of post-traumatic stress symptoms during the course of rehabilitation for whiplash injuries. *Pain, 145*(3), 325–331. http://doi.org/10.1016/j.pain.2009.06.031

Takasaki, H., Chien, C. W., Johnston, V., Treleaven, J., & Jull, G. (2012). Validity and reliability of the perceived deficit questionnaire to assess cognitive symptoms in people with chronic whiplash-associated disorders. *Archives of Physical Medicine and Rehabilitation, 93*(10), 1774–1781. http://doi.org/10.1016/j.apmr.2012.05.013

Tencer, A. F., Mirza, S., & Cummings, P. (2001). Do "whiplash" victims with neck pain differ from those with neck pain and other symptoms? *Annual Proceedings / Association for the Advancement of Automotive Medicine. Association for the Advancement of Automotive Medicine, 45*, 203–214.

Treleaven, J., Jull, G., & Sterling, M. (2003). Dizziness and unsteadiness following whiplash injury: Characteristic features and relationship with cervical joint position error. *Journal of Rehabilitation Medicine, 35*(1), 36–43. http://doi.org/10.1080/16501970306109

Vendrig, A. A., Castro, W. H. M., Scholten-Peeters, G. G. M., & van Akkerveeken, P. F. (2004). Practical guidelines for the prevention of chronic symptoms after a whiplash injury, based on published evidence. *Nederlands*

Tijdschrift Voor Geneeskunde, 148(35), 1716–1720.

Vendrig, A. A., van Akkerveeken, P. F., & McWhorter, K. R. (2000). Results of a multimodal treatment program for patients with chronic symptoms after a whiplash injury of the neck. *Spine, 25*(2), 238–244.

Wallis, B. J., Lord, S. M., Barnsley, L., & Bogduk, N. (1996). Pain and psychologic symptoms of Australian patients with whiplash. *Spine, 21*(7), 804–810. http://doi.org/10.1097/00007632-199604010-00006

Williamson, E., Williams, M. A., Gates, S., & Lamb, S. E. (2014). Risk factors for chronic disability in a cohort of patients with acute whiplash associated disorders seeking physiotherapy treatment for persisting symptoms. *Physiotherapy (United Kingdom)*. http://doi.org/10.1016/j.physio.2014.04.004

Winkelstein, B. A. (2011). How Can Animal Models Inform on the Transition to Chronic Symptoms in Whiplash? *Spine.* http://doi.org/10.1097/BRS.0b013e3182387f96

Whiplash Internet Articles and Research

ACA. (2015). Retrieved on February 2, 2015, from http://www.acatoday.org/content_css.cfm?CID=3131.

Chiropractic Care: Symptoms of Whiplash. (2015). Retrieved on February 2, 2015, from http://www.spineuniverse.com/conditions/whiplash/chiropractic-care-symptoms-whiplash.

Concussion Signs and Symptoms | Axon Sports. (2015). Retrieved on February 2, 2015, from https://www.axonsports.com/index.cfm?pid=82.

Signs and symptoms of whiplash injury. (2015). Retrieved on February 2, 2015, from http://www.the-claim-solicitors.co.uk/whiplash/whiplash-injury-symptoms.htm.

Symptoms of Whiplash are as individual as every accident is unique.. (2015). Retrieved on February 2, 2015, from http://www.chiropractic-help.com/symptoms-of-whiplash.html.

Symptoms of Whiplash. (2015). Retrieved on February 2, 2015, from http://www.rightdiagnosis.com/w/whiplash/symptoms.htm.

What Is Whiplash?. (2015). Retrieved on February 2, 2015, from http://www.spine-health.com/conditions/neck-pain/what-whiplash.

What is whiplash? What causes whiplash?. (2015). Retrieved on February 2, 2015, from http://www.medicalnewstoday.com/articles/174605.php.

Whiplash (medicine). (2015). Retrieved on February 2, 2015, from http://en.wikipedia.org/wiki/Whiplash_(medicine).

Whiplash Associated Disorders. (2015). Retrieved on February 2, 2015, from http://www.physio-pedia.com/Whiplash_Associated_Disorders.

Whiplash Injuries: The Basics | Nolo.com. (2015). Retrieved on February 2, 2015, from http://www.nolo.com/legal-encyclopedia/whiplash-injuries-basics-32286.html.

Whiplash Injury: Pain, Treatment, Symptoms, Causes, and More. (2015). Retrieved on February 2, 2015, from http://www.webmd.com/back-pain/neck-strain-whiplash.

Whiplash Overview, Causes, Symptoms. (2015). Retrieved on February 2, 2015, from http://www.healthcommunities.com/whiplash/causes-symptoms-of-whiplash.shtml.

Whiplash Symptoms and Signs. (2015). Retrieved on February 2, 2015, from http://www.healthguidance.org/entry/12312/1/Whiplash-Symptoms-and-Signs.html.

Whiplash Symptoms. (2015). Retrieved on February 2, 2015, from http://www.car-accident-facts.com/whiplash-symptoms.html.

Whiplash and Cervical Spine Injury | Patient.co.uk. (2015). Retrieved on February 2, 2015, from http://www.patient.co.uk/doctor/whiplash-and-cervical-spine-injury.

Whiplash: Diagnosis, Treatments & Complications. (2015). Retrieved on February 2, 2015, from http://www.healthline.com/health/whiplash.

Whiplash: Get the Facts on Symptoms of this Neck Injury. (2015). Retrieved on February 2, 2015, from http://www.medicinenet.com/whiplash/article.htm.

Whiplash: Symptoms, diagnosis and treatment. (2015). Retrieved on February 2, 2015, from http://www.webmd.boots.com/pain-management/guide/pain-management-whiplash.

Whiplash. (2015). Retrieved on February 2, 2015, from http://www.knowyourback.org/pages/spinalconditions/injuries/whiplash.aspx.

Whiplash. (2015). Retrieved on February 2, 2015, from http://www.nhs.uk/Conditions/Whiplash/Pages/Symptoms.aspx.

vertigo and hearing symptoms after whiplash. (2015). Retrieved on February 2, 2015, from http://www.dizziness-and-balance.com/disorders/post/whiplash.html.

PhysioAdvisor/ Get Started Pty Ltd. (2015). *Neck Whiplash.* Retrieved on February 2, 2015, from http://www.physioadvisor.com.au/9617350/neck-whiplash-whiplash-injury-physioadvisor.htm.

Sturzenegger M , et al.. (2015). *Presenting symptoms and signs after whiplash injury: the influence ....* Retrieved on February 2, 2015, from http://www.ncbi.nlm.nih.gov/pubmed/8164827.

Suissa S , et al.. (2015). *The relation between initial symptoms and signs and the prognosis ....* Retrieved on February 2, 2015, from http://www.ncbi.nlm.nih.gov/pubmed/11276835.

CHAPTER 6
DIAGNOSIS

This Chapter will discuss the concept of diagnosis, including the difference between health conditions that are **misdiagnosed** and those that are **undiagnosed**. This Chapter will also examine the difference between common diagnosis and a differential diagnoses.

The Diagnostic and Differential Diagnostic Process

The term diagnosis refers to the *process* of identifying a disease, based on the signs and symptoms of disease, and a **diagnostic procedure** is a method used to arrive at a diagnosis. Most frequently, doctors base diagnostic determinations on **medical tests** and **observation** to identify a disease or condition. Through test and observation the doctor is attempting to either identify a physical, biological, chemical, emotional, or psychological condition not normally present in a healthy person **OR** one that is present in a healthy person but absent in a person with a particular illness or disease. In this regard, the diagnostic process generally begins with the doctor making an educated guess as to which condition is most likely present, and through tests and observation confirming or denying the presence or absence of disease or illness.

When a doctor fails to diagnosis a disease that is actually present the disease has gone **undiagnosed** and when the doctor determines one disease is present when in fact it is another the health condition is **misdiagnosed**. Obviously, both concepts can go hand-in-hand as the the disease that is present but not identified is undiagnosed and the disease that is identified but not present is misdiagnosed.

On the other hand, a process of **differential diagnosis** is one that, based on the signs and symptoms, a doctor determines that two or more alternative diseases or conditions are nearly equally likely to be present. In essence, the differential diagnostic procedure is a "process of elimination" where a list of possible diseases and disorders is constructed, and possible diseases are removed one-by-one. To eliminate alternative health problems, a physician will use a combination of medical tests, observation, intuition, and past experience to rule-out individual health conditions until only a single condition remains on the list. Because a differential diagnosis attempts to distinguish health disorders that present themselves in a very similar manner, the differential diagnostic process is typically more involved and time-consuming than normal diagnostic protocols. For the same reason and for some conditions, the differential diagnostic process may result in fewer instances of undiagnosed disease but more instances of misdiagnosis.

Medical tests are used to screen for or diagnose health conditions that may be present in a patient or monitor conditions that already exist. **Diagnostic tests** are generally performed only after a patient reports symptoms of a disease or health condition or in response to signs observed by a medical professional. The most methods to diagnose Whiplash are discussed below.

Whiplash Journal Articles

Annis, R. S. (1999). Whiplash Injuries Current Concepts in Prevention, Diagnosis, and Treatment of the Cervical Whiplash Syndrome. *The Journal of the Canadian Chiropractic Association*, *43*(2), 125–126.

Binder, A. (2007). The diagnosis and treatment of nonspecific neck pain and whiplash. *Europa Medicophysica*, *43*(1), 79–89.

Bogduk, N. (2011). On Cervical Zygapophysial Joint Pain After Whiplash. *Spine*. http://doi.org/10.1097/BRS.0b013e3182387f1d

Brault, J. R., Siegmund, G. P., & Wheeler, J. B. (2000). Cervical muscle response during whiplash: Evidence of a lengthening muscle contraction. *Clinical Biomechanics*, *15*(6), 426–435. http://doi.org/10.1016/S0268-0033(99)00097-2

Buitenhuis, J., de Jong, P. J., Jaspers, J. P. C., & Groothoff, J. W. (2006). Relationship between posttraumatic stress disorder symptoms and the course of whiplash complaints. *Journal of Psychosomatic Research*, *61*(5), 681–689. http://doi.org/10.1016/j.jpsychores.2006.07.008

Centre, S. A., & Recovery, I. (2008). Clinical guidelines for best practice management of acute and chronic whiplash-associated disorders. *Injury*, (November), 97. Retrieved from http://espace.library.uq.edu.au/view/UQ:266894

Chen, H., Yang, K. H., & Wang, Z. (2009). Biomechanics of whiplash injury. *Chinese Journal of Traumatology = Zhonghua Chuang Shang Za Zhi / Chinese Medical Association*, *12*(5), 305–314. http://doi.org/10.3760/cma.j.issn.1008-1275.2009.05.011

Côté, P., Cassidy, J. D., Carroll, L., Frank, J. W., & Bombardier, C. (2001). A systematic review of the prognosis of acute whiplash and a new conceptual framework to synthesize the literature. *Spine*, *26*(19), E445–E458. http://doi.org/10.1097/00007632-200110010-00020

Curatolo, M., Bogduk, N., Ivancic, P. C., McLean, S. A., Siegmund, G. P., &

Winkelstein, B. a. (2011). The role of tissue damage in whiplash-associated disorders: discussion paper 1. *Spine*, *36*(25 Suppl), S309–15. http://doi.org/10.1097/BRS.0b013e318238842a

Dommerholt, J. (2005). Persistent myalgia following whiplash. *Current Pain and Headache Reports*, *9*(5), 326–330. http://doi.org/10.1007/s11916-005-0008-5

Epstein, J. B., & Klasser, G. D. (2011). Whiplash-associated disorders and temporomandibular symptoms following motor-vehicle collisions. *Quintessence International (Berlin, Germany : 1985)*, *42*(1), e1–e14.

Ettlin, T. M., Kischka, U., Reichmann, S., Radii, E. W., Heim, S., Wengen, D., & Benson, D. F. (1992). Cerebral symptoms after whiplash injury of the neck: a prospective clinical and neuropsychological study of whiplash injury. *Journal of Neurology, Neurosurgery, and Psychiatry*, *55*(10), 943–948. http://doi.org/10.1136/jnnp.55.10.943

Ettlin, T., Schuster, C., Stoffel, R., Brüderlin, A., & Kischka, U. (2008). A Distinct Pattern of Myofascial Findings in Patients After Whiplash Injury. *Archives of Physical Medicine and Rehabilitation*, *89*(7), 1290–1293. http://doi.org/10.1016/j.apmr.2007.11.041

Freeman, M. D., & Croft, A. C. (1998). The controversy over late whiplash: Are chronic symptoms after whiplash real ? In *Whiplash injuries: Current concepts in prevention, diagnosis, and treatment of the cervical whiplash sndrome* (pp. 161–165).

Freeman, M. D., Croft, A. C., & Rossignol, A. M. (1998). "Whiplash associated disorders: redefining whiplash and its management" by the Quebec Task Force. A critical evaluation. *Spine*, *23*(9), 1043–1049. http://doi.org/10.1097/00007632-199805010-00015

Freitag, P., Greenlee, M. W., Wachter, K., Ettlin, T. M., & Radue, E. W. (2001). fMRI response during visual motion stimulation in patients with late whiplash syndrome. *Neurorehabilitation and Neural Repair*, *15*(1), 31–37. http://doi.org/10.1177/154596830101500105

Gerstenkorn, C., Cacciola, R., Thomusch, O., Brucke, M., Talbot, D., & Dralle, H. Delayed diagnosis of odontoid fracture after whiplash trauma of the cervical spine, 103 Der Unfallchirurg 895–897 (2000).

Greening, J., Dilley, A., & Lynn, B. (2005). In vivo study of nerve movement and mechanosensitivity of the median nerve in whiplash and non-specific arm pain patients. *Pain, 115*(3), 248–253. http://doi.org/10.1016/j.pain.2005.02.023

Hestnes, A. (1997). Whiplash injuries with objective findings. Delayed diagnosis of fractures of the odontoid process. *Tidsskrift for Den Norske Laegeforening : Tidsskrift for Praktisk Medicin, Ny Raekke, 117*(1), 21–22.

HUDDLESTON, O. L. (1958). Whiplash injuries; diagnosis and treatment. *California Medicine, 89*(5), 318–321.

Huddleston, O. L. (1958). WHIPLASH INJURIES—Diagnosis and Treatment. *California Medicine, 89*(5), 318–321.

Keuter, E. J. W., Minderhoud, J. M., Verhagen, A. P., Valk, M., & Rosenbrand, C. J. G. M. K. (2009). The multidisciplinary guideline "Diagnosis and treatment of people with whiplash-associated disorder I or II." *Nederlands Tijdschrift Voor Geneeskunde, 153*, B7.

Krakenes, J., & Kaale, B. R. (2006). Magnetic resonance imaging assessment of craniovertebral ligaments and membranes after whiplash trauma. *Spine, 31*(24), 2820–2826. http://doi.org/10.1097/01.brs.0000245871.15696.1f

Lonnberg, F. (2001). [Whiplash. Epidemiology, diagnosis and treatment]. *Ugeskr Laeger, 163*(16), 2231–2236. Retrieved from http://www.ncbi.nlm.nih.gov/entrez/query.fcgi?cmd=Retrieve&db=PubMed&dopt=Citation&list_uids=11344657

Lønnberg, F. (2001). Whiplash. Epidemiology, diagnosis and treatment. *Ugeskrift for Laeger, 163*(16), 2231–2236.

Ludolph, E., & Meindl, U. The diagnosis of so-called whiplash injury of the cervical vertebrae. A case report, 16 Unfallchirurgie 213–216 (1990).

Martin, J.-L., Pérez, K., Marí-Dell'olmo, M., & Chiron, M. (2008). Whiplash risk estimation based on linked hospital-police road crash data from France and Spain. *Injury Prevention : Journal of the International Society for Child and Adolescent Injury Prevention, 14*(3), 185–190. http://doi.org/10.1136/ip.2007.016600

Muhle, C., Brossmann, J., Biederer, J., Jahnke, T., Grimm, J., & Heller, M. (2002a). [Alar ligaments: radiological aspects in the diagnosis of patients with whiplash injuries]. *Rofo, 174*(4), 416–422. http://doi.org/10.1055/s-2002-25124

Muhle, C., Brossmann, J., Biederer, J., Jahnke, T., Grimm, J., & Heller, M. (2002b). [Alar ligaments: radiological aspects in the diagnosis of patients with whiplash injuries]. *RöFo : Fortschritte Auf Dem Gebiete Der Röntgenstrahlen Und Der Nuklearmedizin, 174*(4), 416–22. http://doi.org/10.1055/s-2002-25124

Muhle, C., Brossmann, J., Biederer, J., Jahnke, T., Grimm, J., & Heller, M. (2002c). Alar ligaments: radiological aspects in the diagnosis of patients with whiplash injuries. *RoFo : Fortschritte Auf Dem Gebiete Der Rontgenstrahlen Und Der Nuklearmedizin, 174*(4), 416–422.

Ostojic, Z., Ostojic, L., & Tripalo, D. (2002). [Standardization of diagnosis and therapy in whiplash injuries of the cervical vertebrae]. *Med Arh, 56*(2), 97–100. Retrieved from http://www.ncbi.nlm.nih.gov/entrez/query.fcgi?cmd=Retrieve&db=PubMed&dopt=Citation&list_uids=12014105

Panjabi, M. M., Cholewicki, J., Nibu, K., Grauer, J. N., Babat, L. B., & Dvorak, J. (1998). Mechanism of whiplash injury. *Clinical Biomechanics, 13*(4-5), 239–249. http://doi.org/10.1016/S0268-0033(98)00033-3

Panjabi, M. M., Cholewicki, J., Nibu, K., Grauer, J. N., Babat, L. B., Dvorak, J., & Bär, H. F. (1998). Biomechanics of whiplash injury. *Der Orthopade, 27*(12), 813–819. http://doi.org/10.3760/cma.j.issn.1008-1275.2009.05.011

Poorbaugh, K., Brismée, J. M., Phelps, V., & Sizer, P. S. (2008). Late Whiplash Syndrome: A clinical science approach to evidence-based diagnosis and management. *Pain Practice, 8*(1), 65–89.

http://doi.org/10.1111/j.1533-2500.2007.00168.x

Radanov, B. P. (2000). [Whiplash injury of the cervical spine--initial evaluation and treatment of late sequelae]. *Ther Umsch*, *57*(12), 716–719.

Rodriquez, A. A., Barr, K. P., & Burns, S. P. (2004). Whiplash: pathophysiology, diagnosis, treatment, and prognosis. *Muscle & Nerve*, *29*(6), 768–781. http://doi.org/10.1002/mus.20060

Rodriquez, A. A., Barr, K. P., & Burns, S. P. (2004). Whiplash: pathophysiology, diagnosis, treatment, and prognosis. *Muscle & Nerve*, *29*(6), 768–781. http://doi.org/10.1002/mus.20060

Rothhaupt, D., & Liebig, K. (1994). Diagnosis, analysis and evaluation of functional disorders of the upper cervical spine within the scope of whiplash injuries with nuclear magnetic resonance tomography. *Der Orthopade*, *23*(4), 278–281.

Schnabel, M., Weber, M., Vassiliou, T., Mann, D., Kirschner, M., Gotzen, L., & Kaluza, G. (2004). Diagnosis and therapy of acute complaints after "whiplash injury" in Germany. Results of a representative survey at surgical and trauma departments in Germany. *Der Unfallchirurg*, *107*(4), 300–306. http://doi.org/10.1007/s00113-004-0740-z

Scholten-Peeters, G. G. M., Bekkering, G. E., Verhagen, A. P., van Der Windt, D. A. W. M., Lanser, K., Hendriks, E. J. M., & Oostendorp, R. A. B. (2002). Clinical practice guideline for the physiotherapy of patients with whiplash-associated disorders. *Spine*, *27*(4), 412–422. http://doi.org/10.1097/00007632-200202150-00018

Sizer, P. S., Poorbaugh, K., & Phelps, V. (2004). Whiplash associated disorders: pathomechanics, diagnosis, and management. *Pain Practice : The Official Journal of World Institute of Pain*, *4*(3), 249–266. http://doi.org/10.1111/j.1533-2500.2004.04310.x

Sjöström, H., Allum, J. H. J., Carpenter, M. G., Adkin, A. L., Honegger, F., & Ettlin, T. (2003). *Trunk sway measures of postural stability during clinical balance tests in patients with chronic whiplash injury symptoms. Spine* (Vol.

28).

Stålnacke, B. M. (2009). Relationship between symptoms and psychological factors five years after whiplash injury. *Journal of Rehabilitation Medicine*, *41*(5), 353–359. http://doi.org/10.2340/16501977-0349

Sterling, M. Physical and psychological aspects of whiplash: important considerations for primary care assessment, part 2--case studies., 14 Manual therapy e8–e12 (2009). http://doi.org/10.1016/j.math.2008.03.004

Sterling, M., Jull, G., Vicenzino, B., & Kenardy, J. (2004). *Characterization of acute whiplash-associated disorders. Spine* (Vol. 29).

Taylor, F. R. (2007). Neck collar, "act-as-usual" or active mobilization for whiplash injury? A randomized parallel-group trial. *Headache*. http://doi.org/10.1111/j.1526-4610.2007.00927.x

Vernon, H., Guerriero, R., Kavanaugh, S., Soave, D., & Puhl, A. (2013). Self-rated disability, fear-avoidance beliefs, nonorganic pain behaviors are important mediators of ranges of active motion in chronic whiplash patients. *Disability and Rehabilitation*, *35*(23), 1954–60. http://doi.org/10.3109/09638288.2013.768302

Welter, F. L., & Berwanger, C. (1998a). Whiplash injuries of the cervical spine. Neurologic contribution to diagnosis. Therapy and expert evaluation. *Der Orthopade*, *27*(12), 834–840.

Welter, F. L., & Berwanger, C. (1998b). Whiplash injury of the cervical spine neurology contribution to diagnosis, therapy and expent evaluations. *Orthopade*, *27*, 834–840. http://doi.org/10.1007/s001320050306

Yadla, S., Ratliff, J. K., & Harrop, J. S. (2008). Whiplash: Diagnosis, treatment, and associated injuries. *Current Reviews in Musculoskeletal Medicine*. http://doi.org/10.1007/s12178-007-9008-x

Whiplash Internet Articles and Research

2012 ICD. (2015). Retrieved on February 2, 2015, from

http://www.icd9data.com/2012/Volume1/800-999/840-848/847/847.0.htm.

Doctor who charged £250 to fix whiplash insurance report with fake .... (2015). Retrieved on February 2, 2015, from http://www.dailymail.co.uk/news/article-2380249/Doctor-charged-250-fix-whiplash-insurance-report-fake-diagnosis-face-disciplinary-hearing.html.

WHIPLASH INJURIES—Diagnosis and Treatment. (2015). Retrieved on February 2, 2015, from http://www.ncbi.nlm.nih.gov/pmc/articles/PMC1512522/.

Whiplash (medicine). (2015). Retrieved on February 2, 2015, from http://en.wikipedia.org/wiki/Whiplash_(medicine).

Whiplash Associated Disorders. (2015). Retrieved on February 2, 2015, from http://www.physio-pedia.com/Whiplash_Associated_Disorders.

Whiplash Definition. (2015). Retrieved on February 2, 2015, from http://www.mayoclinic.org/diseases-conditions/whiplash/basics/definition/con-20033090.

Whiplash Diagnosis, Treatment, Prognosis & Prevention. (2015). Retrieved on February 2, 2015, from http://www.healthcommunities.com/whiplash/diagnosis.shtml.

Whiplash Injuries. (2015). Retrieved on February 2, 2015, from http://www.springer.com/medicine/physical/book/978-88-470-5485-1.

Whiplash Injury: Pain, Treatment, Symptoms, Causes, and More. (2015). Retrieved on February 2, 2015, from http://www.webmd.com/back-pain/neck-strain-whiplash.

Whiplash Neck Sprain | Patient.co.uk. (2015). Retrieved on February 2, 2015, from http://www.patient.co.uk/health/whiplash-neck-sprain.

Whiplash Symptoms, Diagnosis, Treatments and Causes .... (2015). Retrieved on February 2, 2015, from http://www.rightdiagnosis.com/w/whiplash/intro.htm.

Whiplash and Cervical Spine Injury | Patient.co.uk. (2015). Retrieved on February 2, 2015, from http://www.patient.co.uk/doctor/whiplash-and-cervical-spine-injury.

Whiplash and Chiropractic Treatment. How to diagnose and treat a .... (2015). Retrieved on February 2, 2015, from http://www.isischiropractic.co.uk/chiropractic_and_whiplash.html.

Whiplash: Diagnosis, Treatments & Complications. (2015). Retrieved on February 2, 2015, from http://www.healthline.com/health/whiplash.

Whiplash: Get Facts on This Injury. (2015). Retrieved on February 2, 2015, from http://www.emedicinehealth.com/whiplash/article_em.htm.

Whiplash: Get the Facts on Symptoms of this Neck Injury. (2015). Retrieved on February 2, 2015, from http://www.medicinenet.com/whiplash/article.htm.

Whiplash: Neck Trauma and Treatment. (2015). Retrieved on February 2, 2015, from http://www.spineuniverse.com/conditions/whiplash/whiplash-neck-trauma-treatment.

Whiplash: Symptoms, diagnosis and treatment. (2015). Retrieved on February 2, 2015, from http://www.webmd.boots.com/pain-management/guide/pain-management-whiplash.

Whiplash: diagnosis, treatment, and associated injuries. (2015). Retrieved on February 2, 2015, from http://www.ncbi.nlm.nih.gov/pmc/articles/PMC2684148/.

Whiplash. (2015). Retrieved on February 2, 2015, from http://www.nhs.uk/conditions/Whiplash/Pages/Introduction.aspx.

Whiplash. (2015). Retrieved on February 2, 2015, from http://www.pinnaclechiropractic.net/conditions/whiplash/.

Whiplash. (2015). Retrieved on February 2, 2015, from http://www.vancouverspinedoctor.com/whiplash.php.

Rodriquez AA , et al.. (2015). *Whiplash: pathophysiology, diagnosis, treatment, and prognosis.*. Retrieved on February 2, 2015, from http://www.ncbi.nlm.nih.gov/pubmed/15170609.

(2015). *Whiplash: symptoms, diagnosis and treatment.* Retrieved on February 2, 2015, from http://www.mirror.co.uk/features/whiplash-symptoms-diagnosis-and-treatment-4145639.

CHAPTER 7
PATHOPHYSIOLOGY

Understanding Pathophysiology

Pathophysiology is used to describe the changes that occur in the body in response to injury or disease. The term pathophysiology is actually the combination of two words, **pathology** and **physiology**.

The human body constantly works to maintain homeostasis, meaning an internal stability between all the interdependent functions and processes that combine to keep human biological processes functioning in a normal, healthy manner. When activities of the body can not maintain homeostasis, disease ensues. Pathology is the scientific study of disease and pathologists are medical professionals who specialize in diagnosing disease. More specifically, the field of pathology is concerned with identifying the nature and physical origin and course of disease. Within the framework of pathology, the related concept **pathogenesis** focuses exclusively on the origin of disease.

On the other hand, physiology is the branch of biology that studies the physical and chemical functions and processes in living organisms. In this regard, human physiologists research the growth and development requirements of the human body, the absorption and use of nutrients to to fuel energy, and the healthy functioning of organs, tissues, and other anatomical structures. For our purposes, the most important distinction between the fields of human pathology and physiology is the former is concerned with the study of the body in a diseased state and the latter is concerned with the body in a healthy state. Therefore, pathophysiology can be thought of as the study of how disease alters the normal biological and chemical processes in a healthy human body.

Whiplash Journal Articles

Abbassian, A., & Giddins, G. E. (2008). Subacromial impingement in patients with whiplash injury to the cervical spine. *Journal of Orthopaedic Surgery and Research, 3*, 25. http://doi.org/10.1186/1749-799X-3-25

Aceves-Avila, F. J., Ferrari, R., & Ramos-Remus, C. (2004). New insights into culture driven disorders. *Best Practice and Research: Clinical Rheumatology.* http://doi.org/10.1016/j.berh.2004.02.004

Andersen, T. E., Elklit, A., & Vase, L. (2011). The relationship between chronic whiplash-associated disorder and post-traumatic stress: attachment-anxiety may be a vulnerability factor. *European Journal of Psychotraumatology.* http://doi.org/10.3402/ejpt.v2i0.5633

Armstrong, L., & Mcilroy, R. (2012). What is the current evidence for the use of kinesio tape ? A LiterAture review. *SportEX Dynamics, 34*, 24–30.

Barnsley, L., Lord, S., & Bogduk, N. (1994). Whiplash injury. *Pain, 58*(3), 283–307.

Berstad, J. R., Baerum, B., Löchen, E. A., Mogstad, T. E., & Sjaastad, O. (1975). Whiplash: chronic organic brain syndrome without hydrocephalus ex vacuo. *Acta Neurologica Scandinavica, 51*(4), 268–284.

Binder, A. (2007). The diagnosis and treatment of nonspecific neck pain and whiplash. *Europa Medicophysica, 43*(1), 79–89.

Birnbaum, K., Maus, U., & Tacke, J. (2010). Functional cervical MRI within the scope of whiplash injuries: Presentation of a new motion device for the cervical spine. *Surgical and Radiologic Anatomy, 32*(2), 181–188. http://doi.org/10.1007/s00276-009-0557-0

Bodack, M. P., Tunkel, R. S., Marini, S. G., & Nagler, W. (1998). Spinal accessory nerve palsy as a cause of pain after whiplash injury: case report. *J Pain Symptom Manage, 15*(5), 321–328. http://doi.org/S0885-3924(98)00008-6 [pii]

Borchgrevink, G., Smevik, O., Haave, I., Haraldseth, O., Nordby, A., & Lereim, I. (1997). MRI of cerebrum and cervical columna within two days after whiplash neck sprain injury. *Injury, 28*(5-6), 331–335. http://doi.org/10.1016/S0020-1383(97)00027-2

Castro, W. H. M., Meyer, S. J., Becke, M. E. R., Nentwig, C. G., Hein, M. F., Ercan, B. I., ... Du Chesne, A. E. (2001). No stress - No whiplash? Prevalence of "whiplash" symptoms following exposure to a placebo rear-end collision. *International Journal of Legal Medicine, 114*(6), 316–322. http://doi.org/10.1007/s004140000193

Curatolo, M., Bogduk, N., Ivancic, P. C., McLean, S. A., Siegmund, G. P., & Winkelstein, B. a. (2011). The role of tissue damage in whiplash-associated disorders: discussion paper 1. *Spine, 36*(25 Suppl), S309–15. http://doi.org/10.1097/BRS.0b013e318238842a

Elliott, J., Jull, G., Noteboom, J. T., Darnell, R., Galloway, G., & Gibbon, W. W. (2006). Fatty infiltration in the cervical extensor muscles in persistent whiplash-associated disorders: a magnetic resonance imaging analysis. *Spine, 31*(22), E847–E855. http://doi.org/10.1097/01.brs.0000240841.07050.34

Elliott, J. M., Kerry, R., Flynn, T., & Parrish, T. B. (2013). Content not quantity is a better measure of muscle degeneration in whiplash. *Manual Therapy, 18*(6), 578–582. http://doi.org/10.1016/j.math.2013.02.002

Elliott, J. M., Noteboom, J. T., Flynn, T. W., & Sterling, M. (2009). Characterization of acute and chronic whiplash-associated disorders. *The Journal of Orthopaedic and Sports Physical Therapy, 39*(5), 312–323. http://doi.org/10.2519/jospt.2009.2826

Fattori, B., Ursino, F., Cingolani, C., Bruschini, L., Dallan, I., & Nacci, A. (2004). Acupuncture treatment of whiplash injury. *The International Tinnitus Journal, 10*(2), 156–160.

Ferrari, R., & Louw, D. (2011). Correlation between expectations of recovery and injury severity perception in whiplash-associated disorders. *Journal of Zhejiang University. Science. B, 12*(8), 683–686. http://doi.org/10.1631/jzus.B1100097

Ferrari, R., Schrader, H., & Obelieniene, D. (1999). Prevalence of temporomandibular disorders associated with whiplash injury in Lithuania. *Oral Surgery, Oral Medicine, Oral Pathology, Oral Radiology, and Endodontics, 87*(6), 653–657. http://doi.org/S1079-2104(99)70155-1 [pii]

Ferrari, R., & Shorter, E. (2003). From railway spine to whiplash--the recycling of nervous irritation. *Medical Science Monitor : International Medical Journal of Experimental and Clinical Research, 9*(11), HY27–Y37. http://doi.org/3602 [pii]

Friedman, M. H., & Weisberg, J. (2000). The Craniocervical Connection: A Retrospective Analysis of 300 Whiplash Patients with Cervical and Temporomandibular Disorders. *Cranio, 18*(3), 163–167.

Greening, J., Dilley, A., & Lynn, B. (2005). In vivo study of nerve movement and mechanosensitivity of the median nerve in whiplash and non-specific arm pain patients. *Pain, 115*(3), 248–253. http://doi.org/10.1016/j.pain.2005.02.023

Guo, Y., & Jia, L. S. (2011). [Current study and research progress of whiplash injury of cervical vertebrae]. *Zhongguo Gu Shang, 24*(7), 613–615. Retrieved from http://www.ncbi.nlm.nih.gov/pubmed/21870411

Henry, G. K., Gross, H. S., Herndon, C. A., & Furst, C. J. (2000). Nonimpact brain injury: neuropsychological and behavioral correlates with consideration of physiological findings. *Applied Neuropsychology, 7*(2), 65–75. http://doi.org/10.1207/S15324826AN0802_9

Joslin, C. C., Khan, S. N., & Bannister, G. C. (2004). Long-term disability after neck injury. a comparative study. *The Journal of Bone and Joint Surgery. British Volume, 86*(7), 1032–1034. http://doi.org/10.1302/0301-620X.86B7.14633

Kenna, C. J. (1984). The whiplash syndrome. A general practitioner's viewpoint. *Australian Family Physician, 13*(4), 256–258.

Krakenes, J., & Kaale, B. R. (2006). Magnetic resonance imaging assessment of craniovertebral ligaments and membranes after whiplash trauma. *Spine,*

31(24), 2820–2826. http://doi.org/10.1097/01.brs.0000245871.15696.1f

Krakenes, J., Kaale, B. R., Moen, G., Nordli, H., Gilhus, N. E., & Rorvik, J. (2002). MRI assessment of the alar ligaments in the late stage of whiplash injury - A study of structural abnormalities and observer agreement. *Neuroradiology*, *44*(7), 617–624. http://doi.org/10.1007/s00234-002-0799-6

Kwan, O., & Fiel, J. (2002). Critical appraisal of facet joints injections for chronic whiplash. *Medical Science Monitor : International Medical Journal of Experimental and Clinical Research*, *8*(8), RA191–A195. http://doi.org/2656 [pii]

Linnman, C., Appel, L., Fredrikson, M., Gordh, T., Söderlund, A., Långström, B., & Engler, H. (2011). Elevated [11c]-d-deprenyl uptake in chronic whiplash associated disorder suggests persistent musculoskeletal inflammation. *PLoS ONE*, *6*(4). http://doi.org/10.1371/journal.pone.0019182

Nordin, M., Carragee, E. J., Hogg-Johnson, S., Weiner, S. S., Hurwitz, E. L., Peloso, P. M., ... Haldeman, S. (2009). Assessment of Neck Pain and Its Associated Disorders. Results of the Bone and Joint Decade 2000-2010 Task Force on Neck Pain and Its Associated Disorders. *Journal of Manipulative and Physiological Therapeutics*, *32*(2 SUPPL.). http://doi.org/10.1016/j.jmpt.2008.11.016

Omar, N., Alvi, F., & Srinivasan, M. S. (2007). An unusual presentation of whiplash injury: long thoracic and spinal accessory nerve injury. *Eur Spine J*, *16 Suppl 3*, 275–277. http://doi.org/10.1007/s00586-007-0413-z

Oosterveld, W. J., Kortschot, H. W., Kingma, G. G., de Jong, H. A., & Saatci, M. R. (1991). Electronystagmographic findings following cervical whiplash injuries. *Acta Oto-Laryngologica*, *111*(2), 201–205. http://doi.org/10.3109/00016489109137375

Panjabi, M. M. (2006). A hypothesis of chronic back pain: Ligament subfailure injuries lead to muscle control dysfunction. *European Spine Journal*, *15*(5), 668–676. http://doi.org/10.1007/s00586-005-0925-3

Panjabi, M. M., Maak, T. G., Ivancic, P. C., & Ito, S. (2006). Dynamic intervertebral foramen narrowing during simulated rear impact. *Spine*, *31*(5), E128–E134. http://doi.org/10.1097/01.brs.0000201243.81745.ba

Pettersson, K., Hildingsson, C., Toolanen, G., Fagerlund, M., & Björnebrink, J. (1997). Disc pathology after whiplash injury. A prospective magnetic resonance imaging and clinical investigation. *Spine*, *22*(3), 283–287; discussion 288.

Pettersson, K., Kärrholm, J., Toolanen, G., & Hildingsson, C. (1995). Decreased width of the spinal canal in patients with chronic symptoms after whiplash injury. *Spine*, *20*(15), 1664–1667. http://doi.org/10.1097/00007632-199508000-00003

Radanov, B. P., Hirlinger, I., Di Stefano, G., & Valach, L. (1992). Attentional processing in cervical spine syndromes. *Acta Neurologica Scandinavica*, *85*(5), 358–362.

Ronnen, H. R., de Korte, P. J., Brink, P. R., van der Bijl, H. J., Tonino, A. J., & Franke, C. L. (1996). Acute whiplash injury: is there a role for MR imaging?--a prospective study of 100 patients. *Radiology*, *201*(1), 93–96. http://doi.org/10.1148/radiology.201.1.8816527

Scott, S., & Sanderson, P. L. (2002a). Whiplash: a biochemical study of muscle injury. *Eur Spine J*, *11*(4), 389–392. http://doi.org/10.1007/s00586-002-0410-1

Scott, S., & Sanderson, P. L. (2002b). Whiplash: a biochemical study of muscle injury. *European Spine Journal : Official Publication of the European Spine Society, the European Spinal Deformity Society, and the European Section of the Cervical Spine Research Society*, *11*(4), 389–392. http://doi.org/10.1007/s00586-002-0410-1

Scott, S., & Sanderson, P. L. (2002c). Whiplash: a biochemical study of muscle injury. *European Spine Journal*, *11*(4), 389–92. http://doi.org/10.1007/s00586-002-0410-1

Söderlund, A., & Lindberg, P. (2003). Whiplash-associated disorders-- predicting disability from a process-oriented perspective of coping. *Clinical*

Rehabilitation, 17(1), 101–107. http://doi.org/10.1191/0269215503cr566oa

Sterling, M., McLean, S. a, Sullivan, M. J. L., Elliott, J. M., Buitenhuis, J., & Kamper, S. J. (2011). Potential processes involved in the initiation and maintenance of whiplash-associated disorders: discussion paper 3. *Spine, 36*(25 Suppl), S322–9. http://doi.org/10.1097/BRS.0b013e318238853f

Tamaki, T., Saito, N., Node, Y., Sawada, K., & Teramoto, A. (2006). Internal carotid artery stenosis due to atherosclerotic plaque damage after whiplash injury. *Journal of Nippon Medical School = Nippon Ika Daigaku Zasshi, 73*(3), 154–7. Retrieved from http://www.ncbi.nlm.nih.gov/pubmed/16790983

Taylor, J. R. (2002). The pathology of whiplash: Neck sprain. *BC Medical Journal, 44*(5), 252–256. Retrieved from http://www.bcmj.org/print/2900

Tominaga, Y., Ndu, A. B., Coe, M. P., Valenson, A. J., Ivancic, P. C., Ito, S., … Panjabi, M. M. (2006). Neck ligament strength is decreased following whiplash trauma. *BMC Musculoskeletal Disorders, 7*, 103. http://doi.org/10.1186/1471-2474-7-103

Treleaven, J., LowChoy, N., Darnell, R., Panizza, B., Brown-Rothwell, D., & Jull, G. (2008). Comparison of Sensorimotor Disturbance Between Subjects With Persistent Whiplash-Associated Disorder and Subjects With Vestibular Pathology Associated With Acoustic Neuroma. *Archives of Physical Medicine and Rehabilitation, 89*(3), 522–530. http://doi.org/10.1016/j.apmr.2007.11.002

Uehara Benites, M. A., Pérez-Garrigues, H., & Morera Pérez, C. (2009). Expresión clínica de las alteraciones del equilibrio en pacientes con síndrome de latigazo cervical. *Acta Otorrinolaringologica Espanola, 60*(3), 155–159. http://doi.org/10.1016/S0001-6519(09)71224-5

Van Geothem, J. W., Biltjes, I. G. G. M., Van Den Hauwe, L., Parizel, P. M., De Schepper, A. M. A., & Van Goethem, J. W. M. (1996). Whiplash injuries: is there a role for imaging? *European Journal of Radiology, 22 (1)*(1), 30–37. http://doi.org/0720048X9500696N [pii]

Yadla, S., Ratliff, J. K., & Harrop, J. S. (2008). Whiplash: Diagnosis, treatment, and associated injuries. *Current Reviews in Musculoskeletal Medicine.* http://doi.org/10.1007/s12178-007-9008-x

Whiplash Internet Articles and Research

Cervical Sprain and Strain. (2015). Retrieved on February 2, 2015, from http://emedicine.medscape.com/article/306176-overview.

Does inflammation explains the complexity of whiplash associated .... (2015). Retrieved on February 2, 2015, from http://www.paininmotion.be/EN/news-inflammationWAD.html.

Full Text: Stopping Late Whiplash: Which Way to Utopia?. (2015). Retrieved on February 2, 2015, from http://www.jrheum.com/subscribers/08/12/2303.html.

Neuroscience for Kids. (2015). Retrieved on February 2, 2015, from https://faculty.washington.edu/chudler/whiplash.html.

Pathophysiology of Whiplash Associated Disorders: Theories and .... (2015). Retrieved on February 2, 2015, from http://link.springer.com/chapter/10.1007%2F978-88-470-2293-5_7.

The biomechanics of whiplash injury | BC Medical Journal. (2015). Retrieved on February 2, 2015, from http://www.bcmj.org/article/biomechanics-whiplash-injury.

Volume 3, Chapter 32. Retinopathy and Distant Extraocular Trauma. (2015). Retrieved on February 2, 2015, from http://www.eyecalcs.com/DWAN/pages/v3/v3c032.html.

Whiplash (medicine). (2015). Retrieved on February 2, 2015, from http://en.wikipedia.org/wiki/Whiplash_(medicine).

Whiplash Associated Disorders. (2015). Retrieved on February 2, 2015, from http://www.physio-pedia.com/Whiplash_Associated_Disorders.

Whiplash Injuries: A Historical Review. (2015). Retrieved on February 2, 2015, from https://ispub.com/IJN/8/2/8723.

Whiplash and Cervical Spine Injury | Patient.co.uk. (2015). Retrieved on February 2, 2015, from http://www.patient.co.uk/doctor/whiplash-and-cervical-spine-injury.

Whiplash injury. (2015). Retrieved on February 2, 2015, from http://ceaccp.oxfordjournals.org/content/early/2013/11/24/bjaceaccp.mkt052.f

Whiplash: Get the Facts on Symptoms of this Neck Injury. (2015). Retrieved on February 2, 2015, from http://www.medicinenet.com/whiplash/article.htm.

vertigo and hearing symptoms after whiplash. (2015). Retrieved on February 2, 2015, from http://www.dizziness-and-balance.com/disorders/post/whiplash.html.

CBP Seminars. (2015). *Whiplash Injuries: Pathophysiology, Diagnosis, Medical ....* Retrieved on February 2, 2015, from http://www.idealspine.com/pages/AJCC_April_05_whiplash_injuries.htm.

Deepak Vasa - RMIT Publishing - RMIT Training PTY LTD (http://www.informit.com.au). (2015). *Australasian Musculoskeletal Medicine.* Retrieved on February 2, 2015, from http://search.informit.com.au/documentSummary;dn=483923564350867;res=

Rodriquez AA, et al.. (2015). *Whiplash: pathophysiology, diagnosis, treatment, and prognosis..* Retrieved on February 2, 2015, from http://www.ncbi.nlm.nih.gov/pubmed/15170609.

CHAPTER 8
TREATMENT

Once a diagnosis Whiplash has been confirmed, a patient generally begins a treatment regime under the supervision of a doctor or other medical specialist. This Chapter defines the terms **treatment** and **therapy** and discusses the most common treatment protocols for Whiplash.

Treatment and Therapy

The term treatment refers to any method used by a person to remedy a health problem. Treatment can also mean doing nothing at all, often termed to "wath and wait." In medicine, treatment is often referred to as **therapy** and for our purposes the terms treatment and therapy will be used synonymously, both being based on the Greek origin of the word "therapy," to mean "curing or healing."

Treatment or therapy can be applied both to a person's biological being as well to their psychological state. Additionally, treatment can be used to remedy or halt the progression of an existing health condition **(abortive therapy)**, prevent the manifestation of a condition in an otherwise healthy person **(prophylatic therapy)**, or increase the comfort or emotional well-being of a patient when an underlying condition can not be completely eliminated **(palliative therapy)**.

During the course of your research, you will discover that the administration of certain treatments, particularly drug treatments, are often qualified by the terms **indications** and **contraindications**. Indications simply describe the circumstances and conditions that should be present before a particular treatment is administered to a patient. One common indication for drug therapies is that a patient avoid alcohol or refrain from eating for a certain period of time prior to taking a medication. Conversely, a contraindication are circumstances where a treatment should not be administered. For example, some drug treatments or physical therapy activities should not be administered in persons with high blood pressure.

There are two types of contraindications, **relative contraindications** and

absolute contraindications. Relative contraindications occur if caution should be taken when using two or more therapies simultaneously. For therapies with relative contraindications multiple treatments should only be employed if the benefits of using more than one treatment are likely to outweigh the risks. As the term suggests, absolute contraindications means two or more treatments should not be simultaneously administred under any circumstance, as the result could cause death or serious and permanent damage. Obviously, depending on how the treatment instructions are worded some indications for treatment can become contraindications with the addition of words like "not" or "don't."

Unlike indications and contraindications, **side effects** of treatment or therapy refers to any effect in addition to, or on top of, the intended effect of the treatment. The term side effect is most commonly used when referring to drug therapies and while effects can be positive, they are most commonly negative or harmful but seldom cause serious or permanent biological or psychological damage.

Finally, therapies are also referred to as either being **first-line therapies** or **second-line therapies**. Quite simply, first-line therapies refer to the first or preferred treatment options and second-line therapies are commonly employed only when the first-line therapy doesn't produce the desirable outcome or if the patient has other health concerns that make the first-line therapy ill-advised because of complications or contraindications.

Whiplash Journal Articles

Aigner, N., Fialka, C., Radda, C., & Vecsei, V. (2006). Adjuvant laser acupuncture in the treatment of whiplash injuries: A prospective, randomized placebo-controlled trial. *Wiener Klinische Wochenschrift, 118*(3-4), 95–99. http://doi.org/10.1007/s00508-006-0530-4

Amirfeyz, R., Cook, J., Gargan, M., & Bannister, G. (2009). The role of physiotherapy in the treatment of whiplash associated disorders: A prospective study. *Archives of Orthopaedic and Trauma Surgery, 129*(7), 973–977. http://doi.org/10.1007/s00402-008-0803-7

Annis, R. S. (1999). Whiplash Injuries Current Concepts in Prevention, Diagnosis, and Treatment of the Cervical Whiplash Syndrome. *The Journal of the Canadian Chiropractic Association, 43*(2), 125–126.

Binder, A. (2007). The diagnosis and treatment of nonspecific neck pain and whiplash. *Europa Medicophysica, 43*(1), 79–89.

Conlin, A., Bhogal, S., Sequeira, K., & Teasell, R. (2005). Treatment of whiplash-associated disorders - Part I: Noninvasive interventions. *Pain Research and Management.*

Dunne, R. L., Kenardy, J., & Sterling, M. (2012). A Randomized Controlled Trial of Cognitive-behavioral Therapy for the Treatment of PTSD in the Context of Chronic Whiplash. *The Clinical Journal oF Pain.* http://doi.org/10.1097/AJP.0b013e318243e16b

Edebol, H., Ake Bood, S., & Norlander, T. (2008). Chronic whiplash-associated disorders and their treatment using flotation-REST (restricted environmental stimulation technique). *Qualitative Health Research, 18*(4), 480–488. http://doi.org/10.1177/1049732308315109

Fattori, B., Borsari, C., Vannucci, G., Casani, A., Cristofani, R., Bonuccelli, L., & Ghilardi, P. L. (1996). Acupuncture treatment for balance disorders following whiplash injury. *Acupuncture and Electro-Therapeutics Research, 21*(3-4), 207–217. http://doi.org/CN-00652369

Fattori, B., Ursino, F., Cingolani, C., Bruschini, L., Dallan, I., & Nacci, A. (2004). Acupuncture treatment of whiplash injury. *Int Tinnitus J*, *10*(2), 156–160. Retrieved from http://www.ncbi.nlm.nih.gov/entrez/query.fcgi?cmd=Retrieve&db=PubMed&dopt=Citation&list_uids=15732514

Fattori, B., Ursino, F., Cingolani, C., Bruschini, L., Dallan, I., & Nacci, A. (2004). Acupuncture treatment of whiplash injury. *The International Tinnitus Journal*, *10*(2), 156–160.

Fernández-de las Peñas, C. (2005). Dorsal Manipulation in Whiplash Injury Treatment. *Journal of Whiplash & Related Disorders*. http://doi.org/10.1300/J180v03n02_05

Fernández De Las Peñas, C., Palomeque Del Cerro, L., & Fernández Carnero, J. (2005). Manual treatment of post-whiplash injury. *Journal of Bodywork and Movement Therapies*, *9*(2), 109–119. http://doi.org/10.1016/j.jbmt.2004.05.002

Fernandez-de-las-Pen As, J, F.-C., Ap, F., R, L.-V., & Jc, M.-P. (2004). Dorsal manipulation in whiplash injury treatment: A randomized controlled trial. In *Journal of Whiplash Related Disorders* (Vol. 3, pp. 55–72). http://doi.org/10.1300/J180v03n02_05

Ferrantelli, J. R., Harrison, D. E., Harrison, D. D., & Stewart, D. (2005). Conservative treatment of a patient with previously unresponsive whiplash-associated disorders using clinical biomechanics of posture rehabilitation methods. *Journal of Manipulative and Physiological Therapeutics*, *28*(3). http://doi.org/10.1016/j.jmpt.2005.02.006

Freund, B. J., & Schwartz, M. (2000). Treatment of whiplash associated with neck pain with botulinum toxin-A: A pilot study. *Journal of Rheumatology*, *27*(2), 481–484.

Hansen, I., Søgaard, K., Christensen, R., Thomsen, B., Manniche, C., & Juul-Kristensen, B. (2011). Neck exercises, physical and cognitive behavioural-graded activity as a treatment for adult whiplash patients with chronic neck pain: Design of a randomised controlled trial. *BMC Musculoskeletal Disorders*. http://doi.org/10.1186/1471-2474-12-274

Hertz, H., Meng, A., Rabl, V., & Kern, H. (1983a). [Treatment of whiplash injuries of the cervical spine with acupuncture]. *Aktuelle Traumatol, 13*(4), 151–153. Retrieved from http://www.ncbi.nlm.nih.gov/entrez/query.fcgi?cmd=Retrieve&db=PubMed&dopt=Citation&list_uids=6138957

Hertz, H., Meng, A., Rabl, V., & Kern, H. (1983b). Treatment of whiplash injuries of the cervical spine with acupuncture. *Aktuelle Traumatologie, 13*(4), 151–153.

Hijioka, A., Narusawa, K., & Nakamura, T. (2001). Risk factors for long-term treatment of whiplash injury in Japan: Analysis of 400 cases. *Archives of Orthopaedic and Trauma Surgery, 121*(9), 490–493. http://doi.org/10.1007/s004020100284

HUDDLESTON, O. L. (1958). Whiplash injuries; diagnosis and treatment. *California Medicine, 89*(5), 318–321.

Huddleston, O. L. (1958). WHIPLASH INJURIES—Diagnosis and Treatment. *California Medicine, 89*(5), 318–321.

Keuter, E. J. W., Minderhoud, J. M., Verhagen, A. P., Valk, M., & Rosenbrand, C. J. G. M. K. (2009). The multidisciplinary guideline "Diagnosis and treatment of people with whiplash-associated disorder I or II." *Nederlands Tijdschrift Voor Geneeskunde, 153*, B7.

Kirvelä, O. A., & Kotilainen, E. (1999). Successful treatment of whiplash-type injury induced severe pain syndrome with epidural stimulation: A case report. *Pain, 80*(1-2), 441–443. http://doi.org/10.1016/S0304-3959(98)00218-8

Krogstad, B. S., Jokstad, A., Dahl, B. L., & Soboleva, U. (1998). Somatic complaints, psychologic distress, and treatment outcome in two groups of TMD patients, one previously subjected to whiplash injury. *Journal of Orofacial Pain, 12*(2), 136–144.

Lonnberg, F. (2001). [Whiplash. Epidemiology, diagnosis and treatment]. *Ugeskr Laeger, 163*(16), 2231–2236. Retrieved from http://www.ncbi.nlm.nih.gov/entrez/query.fcgi?

cmd=Retrieve&db=PubMed&dopt=Citation&list_uids=11344657

Maxwell, M. (1996). Current physiotherapy treatment for whiplash injury to the neck. *Br J Therapy & Rehab, 3*(7), 391–395. http://doi.org/10.12968/bjtr.1996.3.7.14804

Nijs, J., Van Oosterwijck, J., & De Hertogh, W. (2009). Rehabilitation of chronic whiplash: Treatment of cervical dysfunctions or chronic pain syndrome? *Clinical Rheumatology.* http://doi.org/10.1007/s10067-008-1083-x

Oliveira, A., Gevirtz, R., & Hubbard, D. (2006). A psycho-educational video used in the emergency department provides effective treatment for whiplash injuries. *Spine, 31*(15), 1652–1657. http://doi.org/10.1097/01.brs.0000224172.45828.e3

Peeters, G. G., Verhagen, A. P., de Bie, R. A., & Oostendorp, R. A. (2001). The efficacy of conservative treatment in patients with whiplash injury: a systematic review of clinical trials. *Spine, 26*(4), E64–E73.

Provinciali, L., Baroni, M., Illuminati, L., & Ceravolo, M. G. (1996). *Multimodal treatment to prevent the late whiplash syndrome. Scandinavian journal of rehabilitation medicine* (Vol. 28).

Radanov, B. P. (2000). [Whiplash injury of the cervical spine--initial evaluation and treatment of late sequelae]. *Ther Umsch, 57*(12), 716–719.

Rittig-Rasmussen, B., Kongsted, A., Carstensen, T., Bendix, T., Bach, F. W., & Jensen, T. S. (2010). Treatment of whiplash-associated disorders. *Ugeskrift for Laeger, 172*(24), 1818–1820.

Rodriquez, A. A., Barr, K. P., & Burns, S. P. (2004). Whiplash: pathophysiology, diagnosis, treatment, and prognosis. *Muscle & Nerve, 29*(6), 768–781. http://doi.org/10.1002/mus.20060

Rodriquez, A. A., Barr, K. P., & Burns, S. P. (2004). Whiplash: pathophysiology, diagnosis, treatment, and prognosis. *Muscle & Nerve, 29*(6), 768–781. http://doi.org/10.1002/mus.20060

Rosenfeld, M., Gunnarsson, R., & Borenstein, P. (2000a). *Early intervention in whiplash-associated disorders: a comparison of two treatment protocols. Spine (Phila Pa 1976), 25*(14), 1782–1787. Retrieved from http://www.ncbi.nlm.nih.gov/entrez/query.fcgi?cmd=Retrieve&db=PubMed&dopt=Citation&list_uids=10888946

Rosenfeld, M., Gunnarsson, R., & Borenstein, P. (2000b). *Early intervention in whiplash-associated disorders: a comparison of two treatment protocols. Spine* (Vol. 25).

Scholten-Peeters, G. G. M., Verhagen, A. P., Neeleman-van der Steen, C. W. M., Hurkmans, J. C. A. M., Wams, R. W. A., & Oostendorp, R. A. B. (2003). *Randomized clinical trial of conservative treatment for patients with whiplash-associated disorders: considerations for the design and dynamic treatment protocol. Journal of manipulative and physiological therapeutics* (Vol. 26).

Seferiadis, A., Rosenfeld, M., & Gunnarsson, R. (2004). A review of treatment interventions in whiplash-associated disorders. *European Spine Journal : Official Publication of the European Spine Society, the European Spinal Deformity Society, and the European Section of the Cervical Spine Research Society, 13*(5), 387–397. http://doi.org/10.1007/s00586-004-0709-1

Söderlund, A., & Lindberg, P. An integrated physiotherapy/cognitive-behavioural approach to the analysis and treatment of chronic whiplash associated disorders, WAD., 23 Disability and rehabilitation 436–447 (2001). http://doi.org/10.1080/09638280010008870

Stewart, M. J., Maher, C. G., Refshauge, K. M., Herbert, R. D., & Nicholas, M. K. (2008). Patient and clinician treatment preferences do not moderate the effect of exercise treatment in chronic whiplash-associated disorders. *European Journal of Pain, 12*(7), 879–885. http://doi.org/10.1016/j.ejpain.2007.12.009

Thuile, C., & Walzl, M. (2002). *Evaluation of electromagnetic fields in the treatment of pain in patients with lumbar radiculopathy or the whiplash syndrome. NeuroRehabilitation* (Vol. 17).

Vassiliou, T., Kaluza, G., Putzke, C., Wulf, H., & Schnabel, M. (2006). *Physical therapy and active exercises--an adequate treatment for prevention of late whiplash syndrome? Randomized controlled trial in 200 patients. Pain* (Vol. 124).

Vendrig, A. A., van Akkerveeken, P. F., & McWhorter, K. R. (2000). Results of a multimodal treatment program for patients with chronic symptoms after a whiplash injury of the neck. *Spine, 25*(2), 238–244.

Vendrig, L. (1997). Cognitive-behavioral treatment of chronic complaints after whiplash injury of the neck: An explanation. [Dutch]. *Gedragstherapie, 30*(1), 33.

Verhagen, A. P., Peeters, G. G., de Bie, R. A., & Oostendorp, R. A. (2001). Conservative treatment for whiplash. *Cochrane Database of Systematic Reviews (Online)*, (4), CD003338. http://doi.org/10.1002/14651858.CD003338

Vikne, J., Oedegaard, A., Laerum, E., Ihlebaek, C., & Kirkesola, G. (2007). A randomized study of new sling exercise treatment vs traditional physiotherapy for patients with chronic whiplash-associated disorders with unsettled compensation claims. *Journal of Rehabilitation Medicine, 39*(3), 252–259. http://doi.org/10.2340/16501977-0049

Wallis, B. J., Lord, S. M., & Bogduk, N. (1997). Resolution of psychological distress of whiplash patients following treatment by radiofrequency neurotomy: A randomised, double-blind, placebo-controlled trial. *Pain, 73*(1), 15–22. http://doi.org/10.1016/S0304-3959(97)00060-2

WJ, B., & MA, T. (2000). Manual medicine treatment of the cervical spine and whiplash injury. *PHYSICAL MEDICINE REHABILITATION: STATE OF THE ART REVIEWS, 14*(1), 73. Retrieved from http://search.ebscohost.com/login.aspx?direct=true&db=amed&AN=0012176&site=ehost-live

Woodward, M. N., Cook, J. C. H., Gargan, M. F., & Bannister, G. C. (1996). Chiropractic treatment of chronic "whiplash" injuries. *Injury, 27*(9), 643–645. http://doi.org/10.1016/S0020-1383(96)00096-4

Yadla, S., Ratliff, J. K., & Harrop, J. S. (2008). Whiplash: Diagnosis, treatment, and associated injuries. *Current Reviews in Musculoskeletal Medicine.* http://doi.org/10.1007/s12178-007-9008-x

Whiplash Internet Articles and Research

ACA. (2015). Retrieved on February 2, 2015, from http://www.acatoday.org/content_css.cfm?CID=3131.

Chiropractic Treatments for Whiplash. (2015). Retrieved on February 2, 2015, from http://www.spine-health.com/treatment/chiropractic/chiropractic-treatments-whiplash.

How to Treat Whiplash: 8 Steps (with Pictures). (2015). Retrieved on February 2, 2015, from http://www.wikihow.com/Treat-Whiplash.

J.K. Simmons gets the . (2015). Retrieved on February 2, 2015, from http://www.cbsnews.com/news/j-k-simmons-gets-whiplash-treatment-in-snl-promos/.

NINDS Whiplash Information Page. (2015). Retrieved on February 2, 2015, from http://www.ninds.nih.gov/disorders/whiplash/whiplash.htm.

Pain education video appears effective in whiplash treatment. (2015). Retrieved on February 2, 2015, from http://www.apa.org/monitor/feb07/pain.aspx.

UQ Whiplash Evidence Based Resource. (2015). Retrieved on February 2, 2015, from http://www.som.uq.edu.au/whiplash/whiplash-treatments/whiplash-treatment-table.aspx.

Whiplash Associated Disorders. (2015). Retrieved on February 2, 2015, from http://www.physio-pedia.com/Whiplash_Associated_Disorders.

Whiplash Causes, Symptoms, Treatment. (2015). Retrieved on February 2, 2015, from http://www.emedicinehealth.com/whiplash/page5_em.htm.

Whiplash Definition. (2015). Retrieved on February 2, 2015, from http://www.mayoclinic.org/diseases-conditions/whiplash/basics/definition/con-20033090.

Whiplash Injury: Pain, Treatment, Symptoms, Causes, and More. (2015). Retrieved on February 2, 2015, from http://www.webmd.com/back-pain/neck-strain-whiplash.

Whiplash Neck Sprain | Patient.co.uk. (2015). Retrieved on February 2, 2015, from http://www.patient.co.uk/health/whiplash-neck-sprain.

Whiplash Treatment Center LLC. (2015). Retrieved on February 2, 2015, from http://www.yelp.com/biz/whiplash-treatment-center-llc-westminster-2.

Whiplash Treatment: First Aid Information for Whiplash. (2015). Retrieved on February 2, 2015, from http://www.webmd.com/first-aid/whiplash-treatment.

Whiplash: Diagnosis, Treatments & Complications. (2015). Retrieved on February 2, 2015, from http://www.healthline.com/health/whiplash.

Whiplash: Get the Facts on Symptoms of this Neck Injury. (2015). Retrieved on February 2, 2015, from http://www.medicinenet.com/whiplash/article.htm.

Whiplash: Neck Trauma and Treatment. (2015). Retrieved on February 2, 2015, from http://www.spineuniverse.com/conditions/whiplash/whiplash-neck-trauma-treatment.

Whiplash: Symptoms, diagnosis and treatment. (2015). Retrieved on February 2, 2015, from http://www.webmd.boots.com/pain-management/guide/pain-management-whiplash.

Whiplash. (2015). Retrieved on February 2, 2015, from http://www.knowyourback.org/pages/spinalconditions/injuries/whiplash.aspx.

Whiplash. (2015). Retrieved on February 2, 2015, from http://www.netdoctor.co.uk/diseases/facts/whiplash.htm.

Whiplash. (2015). Retrieved on February 2, 2015, from http://www.nhs.uk/Conditions/Whiplash/Pages/Treatment.aspx.

Chicago Tribune. (2015). *How does 'Whiplash' treat jazz?*. Retrieved on February 2, 2015, from http://www.chicagotribune.com/entertainment/music/reich/ct-jazz-whiplash-20141021-column.html.

Conlin A , et al.. (2015). *Treatment of whiplash*. Retrieved on February 2, 2015, from http://www.ncbi.nlm.nih.gov/pubmed/15782244.

PhysioAdvisor/ Get Started Pty Ltd. (2015). *Neck Whiplash*. Retrieved on February 2, 2015, from http://www.physioadvisor.com.au/9617350/neck-whiplash-whiplash-injury-physioadvisor.htm.

Rosenfeld M , et al.. (2015). *Early intervention in whiplash*. Retrieved on February 2, 2015, from http://www.ncbi.nlm.nih.gov/pubmed/10888946.

CHAPTER 9
PROGNOSIS

Defining Prognosis

A prognosis is a forecast as to the probable outcome or status of a disease or health condition at a defined point in time in the future. It is most often used to refer to the estimated chance of survival or recovery, though it can also refer to the chances of complications, the time to recovery, or other probable or possible outcomes.

While a prognosis is most frequently phrased in percentage terms, "the patient with Disease X has a 85% chance of survival," it is ultimately only an opinion made by a doctor, even though the doctor refers to medical research of past outcomes for similarly situated patients to form his opinion. In Biomedical Research, making generalizations about patient prognoses is steeped heavily not only in the biological sciences but in mathematical science and statistics as well, in a field known as "Survival Analysis."

Survival analysis can be defined as a group of statistical methods used to analyze and evaluate data to determine the time to the occurrence of an event. When applied to medicine, the event occurrence, or outcome variable, can be death, the onset a disease, the time necessary for a therapy to be effective, the progression of symptoms, and so forth. Typically, this analytic procedure is performed as part of a larger medical study of a representative sample of patients. In survival analysis data collection is quite straightforward and simply involves observing a patient over time and recording relevant information about the patient at specified intervals.

Once all data is collected, a form of regression analysis (most often the Cox Proportional Hazards Regression model) can be performed. Regression analysis evaluates the change in one or more variables (dependent variables) based on the presence of a second variable or set of variables (independent variables). In survival analysis the independent variable is commonly the presence of a disease or health condition and dependent variables almost always include both an event status (whether an event did or did not occur) and the time to occurrence of the event. A simple example is predicting the time to death for individuals with inoperable lung cancer. In this case the independent variable is the presence of lung cancer and the dependent variables could be death (the event occurrence) and the number of days or years (time) to the death event. Based on the amount of data collected, survival analysis can also get much more specific by making separate determinations based on patient gender, age, the introduction of specific therapies, etc. To account for unique study cases, such as patients who don't die during the duration of the study period or patients who leave a study before death, a special estimator known as the Kaplan-Meier estimator is used to allow researchers to include these cases in study data but still make certain estimates are accurate.

Therefore, a prognosis simply puts in percentage terms the most likely outcome for a patient based on specific factors or variables but does not necessarily mean the event occurrence will occur in every case or, when it does, in the exact time period identified in the prognosis. Remember the research to determine a prognosis is based on hundreds and even thousands of unique cases for unique individuals and is generally only a statement of the most common outcome for the majority, or even plurality, of participants in the study. Put simply then, not all participants likely experienced the same outcome. For this reason, doctors are often hesitant to provide patients with a concrete prognosis since for some diseases and/or the unique characteristics of an individual patient actual outcomes can vary substantially from a common prognosis. This is especially true when research demonstrates multiple potential outcomes are possible. This concept is most clearly illustrated when individuals or the popular media declare a positive outcome of a disease to be a "medical miracle" even though a doctor may deem the same outcome well within the range of medical possibilities. Conversely, absent medical error, negative outcomes when compared to the prognosis given have also become the basis for countless unsuccessful lawsuits claiming medical malpractice.

Whiplash Journal Articles

Bohman, T., Côté, P., Boyle, E., Cassidy, J. D., Carroll, L. J., & Skillgate, E. (2012). Prognosis of patients with whiplash-associated disorders consulting physiotherapy: development of a predictive model for recovery. *BMC Musculoskeletal Disorders, 13*(1), 264. http://doi.org/10.1186/1471-2474-13-264

Bonnier, C., Nassogne, M. C., & Evrard, P. (1995). Outcome and prognosis of whiplash shaken infant syndrome; late consequences after a symptom-free interval. *Developmental Medicine and Child Neurology, 37*(11), 943–956. http://doi.org/10.1016/0887-8994(94)90203-8

Borenstein, P., Rosenfeld, M., & Gunnarsson, R. (2010). Cognitive symptoms, cervical range of motion and pain as prognostic factors after whiplash trauma. *Acta Neurologica Scandinavica, 122*(4), 278–285. http://doi.org/10.1111/j.1600-0404.2009.01305.x

Bramsen, I., & Roelofs, P. (2009). Using the term "whiplash" has no decisive influence for the prognosis: statistical misinterpretation. *Nederlands Tijdschrift Voor Geneeskunde, 153*, A865.

Carroll, L. J., Cassidy, J. D., & Côté, P. (2006). The role of pain coping strategies in prognosis after whiplash injury: Passive coping predicts slowed recovery. *Pain, 124*(1-2), 18–26. http://doi.org/10.1016/j.pain.2006.03.012

Cassidy, J. D., Carroll, L. J., Côté, P., Lemstra, M., Berglund, A., & Nygren, A. (2000). Effect of eliminating compensation for pain and suffering on the outcome of insurance claims for whiplash injury. *The New England Journal of Medicine, 342*(16), 1179–1186. http://doi.org/10.1056/NEJM200004203421606

Centre, S. A., & Recovery, I. (2008). Clinical guidelines for best practice management of acute and chronic whiplash-associated disorders. *Injury*, (November), 97. Retrieved from http://espace.library.uq.edu.au/view/UQ:266894

Cobo, E. P., Mesquida, M. E. P., Fanegas, E. P., Atanasio, E. M., Pastor, M.

B. S., Pont, C. P., ... Cano, L. G. (2010). What factors have influence on persistence of neck pain after a whiplash? *Spine, 35*(9), E338–E343. http://doi.org/10.1097/BRS.0b013e3181c9b075

Côté, P., Cassidy, J. D., & Carroll, L. (2003). The epidemiology of neck pain: what we have learned from our population-based studies. *The Journal of the Canadian Chiropractic Association, 47*(4), 284–290.

Cote, P., Cassidy, J. D., Carroll, L., Frank, J. W., & Bombardier, C. (2001). A systematic review of the prognosis of acute whiplash and a new conceptual framework to synthesize the literature.[see comment]. *Spine, 26*(19), E445–58.

Côté, P., Cassidy, J. D., Carroll, L., Frank, J. W., & Bombardier, C. (2001). A systematic review of the prognosis of acute whiplash and a new conceptual framework to synthesize the literature. *Spine, 26*(19), E445–E458. http://doi.org/10.1097/00007632-200110010-00020

Crutebo, S., Nilsson, C., Skillgate, E., & Holm, L. W. (2010). The course of symptoms for whiplash-associated disorders in Sweden: 6-month followup study. *Journal of Rheumatology, 37*(7), 1527–1533. http://doi.org/10.3899/jrheum.091321

Curtis, P., Spanos, A., & Reid, A. (1995). Persistent symptoms after whiplash injuries implications for prognosis and management. *Journal of Clinical Rheumatology : Practical Reports on Rheumatic & Musculoskeletal Diseases, 1*(3), 149–157. http://doi.org/10.1097/00124743-199506000-00004

Daenen, L., Nijs, J., Raadsen, B., Roussel, N., Cras, P., & Dankaerts, W. (2013). Cervical motor dysfunction and its predictive value for long-term recovery in patients with acute whiplash-associated disorders: a systematic review. *Journal of Rehabilitation Medicine : Official Journal of the UEMS European Board of Physical and Rehabilitation Medicine, 45*(2), 113–22. http://doi.org/10.2340/16501977-1091

Evans, R. W. (1992). Some observations on whiplash injuries.\n(prognosis-pre-existing.../& other studies). *Neurologic Clinics, 10*(4), 975–97. Retrieved from http://www.ncbi.nlm.nih.gov/pubmed/1435666

Fernandez, C. E., Amiri, A., Jaime, J., & Delaney, P. (2009). The relationship of whiplash injury and temporomandibular disorders: a narrative literature review. *Journal of Chiropractic Medicine*. http://doi.org/10.1016/j.jcm.2009.07.006

Ferrari, R. (2010). Predicting central sensitisation: Whiplash patients. *Australian Family Physician*, *39*(11), 863–866.

Freeman, M. D., Croft, A. C., & Rossignol, A. M. (1998). "Whiplash associated disorders: redefining whiplash and its management" by the Quebec Task Force. A critical evaluation. *Spine*, *23*(9), 1043–1049. http://doi.org/10.1097/00007632-199805010-00015

Harder, S., Veilleux, M., & Suissa, S. (1998). The effect of sociodemographic and crash-related factors on the prognosis of whiplash. *Journal of Clinical Epidemiology*, *51*(5), 377–384. http://doi.org/10.1016/S0895-4356(98)00011-0

Hartling, L., Pickett, W., & Brison, R. J. (2002). Derivation of a clinical decision rule for whiplash associated disorders among individuals involved in rear-end collisions. *Accident Analysis and Prevention*, *34*(4), 531–539. http://doi.org/10.1016/S0001-4575(01)00051-3

Holm, L. W., Carroll, L. J., Cassidy, J. D., Skillgate, E., & Ahlbom, A. (2008). Expectations for recovery important in the prognosis of whiplash injuries. *PLoS Medicine*, *5*(5), 0760–0767. http://doi.org/10.1371/journal.pmed.0050105

Juan, F. J. (2004). Use of botulinum toxin-A for musculoskeletal pain in patients with whiplash associated disorders [ISRCTN68653575]. *BMC Musculoskeletal Disorders*, *5*, 5. http://doi.org/10.1186/1471-2474-5-5

Khan, S., Bannister, G., Gargan, M., Asopa, V., & Edwards, A. (2000). Prognosis following a second whiplash injury. *Injury*, *31*(4), 249–251. http://doi.org/10.1016/S0020-1383(99)00291-0

Kivioja, J., Jensen, I., & Lindgren, U. (2005). Early coping strategies do not influence the prognosis after whiplash injuries. *Injury*, *36*(8), 935–940.

http://doi.org/10.1016/j.injury.2004.09.038

Krakenes, J., & Kaale, B. R. (2006). Magnetic resonance imaging assessment of craniovertebral ligaments and membranes after whiplash trauma. *Spine*, *31*(24), 2820–2826. http://doi.org/10.1097/01.brs.0000245871.15696.1f

M, R., A, S., J, C., & R, G. (2003). Active intervention in patients with whiplash-associated disorders improves long-term prognosis: a randomized controlled clinical trial. In *Spine* (Vol. 28, pp. 2491–2498). Retrieved from http://www.mrw.interscience.wiley.com/cochrane/clcentral/articles/959/CN-00474959/frame.html

Milicic, A., Jovanovic, A., Milankov, M., Savic, D., & Stankovic, M. (1994). [Evaluation of long-term prognosis in patients with whiplash syndrome]. *Med Pregl*, *47*(9-10), 341–343. Retrieved from http://www.ncbi.nlm.nih.gov/entrez/query.fcgi?cmd=Retrieve&db=PubMed&dopt=Citation&list_uids=7565324

Milicić, A., Jovanović, A., Milankov, M., Savić, D., & Stanković, M. (1994). Evaluation of long-term prognosis in patients with whiplash syndrome. *Medicinski Pregled*, *47*(9-10), 341–343.

Olivegren, H., Jerkvall, N., Hagström, Y., & Carlsson, J. (1999). The long-term prognosis of whiplash-associated disorders (WAD). *European Spine Journal*, *8*(5), 366–370. http://doi.org/10.1007/s005860050189

Pujol, A., Puig, L., Mansilla, J., & Idiaquez, I. (2003). Relevant factors in medico-legal prognosis of whiplash injury. *Medicina Clinica*, *121*(6), 209–215. http://doi.org/13049926 [pii]

Rodriquez, A. A., Barr, K. P., & Burns, S. P. (2004). Whiplash: pathophysiology, diagnosis, treatment, and prognosis. *Muscle & Nerve*, *29*(6), 768–781. http://doi.org/10.1002/mus.20060

Rodriquez, A. A., Barr, K. P., & Burns, S. P. (2004). Whiplash: pathophysiology, diagnosis, treatment, and prognosis. *Muscle & Nerve*, *29*(6), 768–781. http://doi.org/10.1002/mus.20060

Rosenfeld, M., Seferiadis, A., Carlsson, J., & Gunnarsson, R. (2003). Active intervention in patients with whiplash-associated disorders improves long-term prognosis - A randomized controlled clinical trial. *SPINE*, *28*(22), 2491–2498. http://doi.org/10.1097/01.BRS.0000090822.96814.13

Rosenfeld, M., Seferiadis, A., Carlsson, J., & Gunnarsson, R. (2003). *Active intervention in patients with whiplash-associated disorders improves long-term prognosis: a randomized controlled clinical trial. Spine* (Vol. 28).

Scholten-Peeters, G. G. M., Bekkering, G. E., Verhagen, A. P., van Der Windt, D. A. W. M., Lanser, K., Hendriks, E. J. M., & Oostendorp, R. A. B. (2002). Clinical practice guideline for the physiotherapy of patients with whiplash-associated disorders. *Spine*, *27*(4), 412–422. http://doi.org/10.1097/00007632-200202150-00018

Sterling, M. Physical and psychological aspects of whiplash: important considerations for primary care assessment, part 2--case studies., 14 Manual therapy e8–e12 (2009). http://doi.org/10.1016/j.math.2008.03.004

Sterling, M., Carroll, L. J., Kasch, H., Kamper, S. J., & Stemper, B. (2011a). Prognosis after whiplash injury: where to from here? Discussion paper 4. *Spine (Phila Pa 1976)*, *36*(25 Suppl), S330–4. http://doi.org/10.1097/BRS.0b013e3182388523

Sterling, M., Carroll, L. J., Kasch, H., Kamper, S. J., & Stemper, B. (2011a). Prognosis after whiplash injury: where to from here? Discussion paper 4. *Spine*, *36*(25 Suppl), S330–4. http://doi.org/10.1097/BRS.0b013e3182388523

Sterling, M., Carroll, L. J., Kasch, H., Kamper, S. J., & Stemper, B. (2011b). Prognosis after whiplash injury: where to from here? Discussion paper 4. *Spine (Phila Pa 1976)*, *36*(25 Suppl), S330–4. http://doi.org/10.1097/BRS.0b013e3182388523

Sterling, M., Carroll, L. J., Kasch, H., Kamper, S. J., & Stemper, B. (2011b). Prognosis Following Whiplash Injury: Where to From Here? *Spine (Phila Pa 1976)*. http://doi.org/10.1097/BRS.0b013e3182388523

Sterling, M., Jull, G., & Kenardy, J. (2006). Physical and psychological factors maintain long-term predictive capacity post-whiplash injury. *Pain*, *122*(1-2), 102–108. http://doi.org/10.1016/j.pain.2006.01.014

Sterling, M., & Kenardy, J. (2008). Physical and psychological aspects of whiplash: Important considerations for primary care assessment. *Manual Therapy*, *13*(2), 93–102. http://doi.org/10.1016/j.math.2007.11.003

Storaci, R., Manelli, A., Schiavone, N., Mangia, L., Prigione, G., & Sangiorgi, S. (2006). Whiplash injury and oculomotor dysfunctions: Clinical-posturographic correlations. *European Spine Journal*, *15*(12), 1811–1816. http://doi.org/10.1007/s00586-006-0085-0

Suissa, S. (2003). Risk factors of poor prognosis after whiplash injury. *Pain Res Manag*, *8*(2), 69–75. Retrieved from http://www.ncbi.nlm.nih.gov/entrez/query.fcgi?cmd=Retrieve&db=PubMed&dopt=Citation&list_uids=12879136

Suissa, S. (2003a). Risk factors of poor prognosis after whiplash injury. *Pain Research & Management : The Journal of the Canadian Pain Society = Journal de La Société Canadienne Pour Le Traitement de La Douleur*, *8*(2), 69–75. Retrieved from http://www.ncbi.nlm.nih.gov/pubmed/12879136

Suissa, S. (2003b). Risk factors of poor prognosis after whiplash injury. *Pain Research & Management : The Journal of the Canadian Pain Society = Journal de La Societe Canadienne Pour Le Traitement de La Douleur*, *8*(2), 69–75.

Suissa, S., Harder, S., & Veilleux, M. (2001). The relation between initial symptoms and signs and the prognosis of whiplash. *European Spine Journal*, *10*(1), 44–49. http://doi.org/10.1007/s005860000220

Treleaven, J. (2011). Dizziness, Unsteadiness, Visual Disturbances, and Postural Control. *Spine*. http://doi.org/10.1097/BRS.0b013e3182387f78

Verhagen, A. P., Lewis, M., Schellingerhout, J. M., Heymans, M. W., Dziedzic, K., de Vet, H. C. W., & Koes, B. W. (2011). Do whiplash patients differ from other patients with non-specific neck pain regarding pain, function or prognosis? *Manual Therapy*, *16*(5), 456–462.

http://doi.org/10.1016/j.math.2011.02.009

Walton, D. M., Pretty, J., MacDermid, J. C., & Teasell, R. W. (2009). Risk factors for persistent problems following whiplash injury: results of a systematic review and meta-analysis. *The Journal of Orthopaedic and Sports Physical Therapy, 39*(5), 334–350. http://doi.org/10.2519/jospt.2009.2765

Whiplash Internet Articles and Research

Clinical guidelines for best practice management of acute and .... (2015). Retrieved on February 2, 2015, from http://www.nhmrc.gov.au/guidelines-publications/cp112.

Diagnosis and prognosis of whiplash injury. (2015). Retrieved on February 2, 2015, from http://www.the-claim-solicitors.co.uk/whiplash/diagnosis-and-prognosis-of-whiplash-injury.htm.

Expectations for Recovery Important in the Prognosis of Whiplash .... (2015). Retrieved on February 2, 2015, from http://www.plosmedicine.org/article/info:doi/10.1371/journal.pmed.0050105.

Factors Affecting the Whiplash Injury. (2015). Retrieved on February 2, 2015, from http://www.spine-health.com/conditions/neck-pain/factors-affecting-whiplash-injury.

Full Text: Whiplash: Social Interventions and Solutions. (2015). Retrieved on February 2, 2015, from https://jrheum.com/subscribers/08/12/2300.html.

NINDS Whiplash Information Page. (2015). Retrieved on February 2, 2015, from http://www.ninds.nih.gov/disorders/whiplash/whiplash.htm.

Prognosis of Whiplash. (2015). Retrieved on February 2, 2015, from http://www.rightdiagnosis.com/w/whiplash/prognosis.htm.

Prognosis of patients with whiplash. (2015). Retrieved on February 2, 2015, from http://www.biomedcentral.com/1471-2474/13/264.

Risk Factors for Persistent Problems Following Whiplash Injury .... (2015).

Retrieved on February 2, 2015, from
http://www.jospt.org/doi/pdf/10.2519/jospt.2009.2765.

The relation between initial symptoms and signs and the prognosis .... (2015). Retrieved on February 2, 2015, from
http://link.springer.com/content/pdf/10.1007/s005860000220.pdf.

The role of pain coping strategies in prognosis after whiplash injury .... (2015). Retrieved on February 2, 2015, from
http://www.sciencedirect.com/science/article/pii/S0304395906001631.

Whiplash (medicine). (2015). Retrieved on February 2, 2015, from
http://en.wikipedia.org/wiki/Whiplash_(medicine).

Whiplash Associated Disorders. (2015). Retrieved on February 2, 2015, from
http://www.physio-pedia.com/Whiplash_Associated_Disorders.

Whiplash Diagnosis, Treatment, Prognosis & Prevention. (2015). Retrieved on February 2, 2015, from
http://www.healthcommunities.com/whiplash/diagnosis.shtml.

Whiplash and Cervical Spine Injury | Patient.co.uk. (2015). Retrieved on February 2, 2015, from http://www.patient.co.uk/doctor/whiplash-and-cervical-spine-injury.

Whiplash. (2015). Retrieved on February 2, 2015, from
http://www.nhs.uk/Conditions/Whiplash/Pages/Treatment.aspx.

CBP Seminars. (2015). *Whiplash Injuries: Pathophysiology, Diagnosis, Medical ....* Retrieved on February 2, 2015, from
http://www.idealspine.com/pages/AJCC_April_05_whiplash_injuries.htm.

Suissa S. (2015). *Risk factors of poor prognosis after whiplash injury..* Retrieved on February 2, 2015, from
http://www.ncbi.nlm.nih.gov/pubmed/12879136.

anonymous. (2015). *Whiplash | Spine Center | NYU Langone Medical Center | New York.* Retrieved on February 2, 2015, from

http://hjd.med.nyu.edu/spine/patient-education/spine-problems/neck-and-arm-pain/whiplash.

faculty of medicine. (2015). *Bedside Clinical Tests of Prognosis Following Whiplash Injury*. Retrieved on February 2, 2015, from http://www1.imperial.ac.uk/msklab/archives/whiplashinjury/.

CHAPTER 10
APPLIED RESEARCH & RESOURCES

This final chapter provides additional resources for the reader interested in examining Whiplash from a different or more in-depth perspective. Increasingly, mainstream medical researchers and doctors are recognizing how important nutrition, alternative treatments, and other so-called fringe therapies can be in preventing and treating disease. This chapter briefly provides context to these emerging therapies and identifies the best resources available for further study. Likewise, this chapter discusses additional research sources for those seeking additional information about applied research, namely information resources for those interested in the role of pharmaceuticals and biotechnology in treating disease and health conditions. Finally, this chapter provides a primer on finding and researching professional journals and other similar written publications.

Alternative Health & Complementary Medicine

More than 40% of all Americans use some form of complementary, alternative, or integrative medicine. While similar, each of these three (3) medical treatment types has a distinct meaning.

Complementary Medicine means using a non-mainstream medical approach in conjunction with conventional medicine, separating each into its own treatment. **Alternative Medicine** is when a non-mainstream medical approach is used in place or instead of a conventional approach. **Integrative Medicine** is combining a non-mainstream approach with conventional medicine to construct one unfied treatment treatment protocol.

Regardless of the exact approach, for our purposes we will describe all three together under the term Alternative Medicine. To further understand this non-mainstream medical approach it worthwhile to note that most alternative therapies have two (2) First, is the use of all natural products like herbs (botanicals), vitamins, and minerals and are collectively marketed as dietary supplements. In the past several years interest in dietary supplements has increased dramatically. The most popular supplements in recent years include fish oil and other omega 3s, ginko biloba, and echinacea. A second hallmark of most alternative medicine methods is the focus on mind and body practices. Common mind and body alternative therapies include acupuncture, massage therapy, movement therapies (like pilates), meditation, and relaxation therapies accomplished through breathing exercise, muscle relaxation, or guided imagery.

While alternative therapies were once dismissed by licensed physicians in recent years it has rapidly received more acceptance in conventional Western medicine and has become increasingly commonplace for treatment of a large number health conditions.

National Center for Complementary and Alternative Medicine (NCCAM)

The National Center for Complementary and Alternative Medicine (NCCAM) researches alternative medical therapies and is an agency within the larger National Institutes of Health. The NCCAM research database allows users to search for medical research related to specific health conditions and alternative medicine at http://nccam.nih.gov/health/atoz.htm. To perform a search simply enter your keywords in the search box and select "Search" or use the index of health topics located on the same page.

Nutrition

Doctors have long recognized the association between good nutrition and good health. Nutrition is the science of foods and nutrients contained in food. Nutrients found in food are used by the body to support growth, provide energy, and maintain and support body tissue. Thus, the study of nutrition examines the relationship between diet and health, including the relationship between diet and disease. Examples of chronic health conditions commonly associated with nutrition include Cardiovascular Disease, Obesity, Type II Diabetes, Osteoporosis, and Hypertension.

National Institutes of Health Office of Dietary Supplements (ODS)

The National Institutes of Health Office of Dietary Supplements (ODS) is an office of the National Institutes of Health and provides users a searchable database containing bibliographic information about nutrition and health and disease. The database, called the International Bibliographic Information on Dietary Supplements, or IBIDS for short can be accessed free of charge at http://ods.od.nih.gov/Health_Information/IBIDS.aspx.

The IBIDS database is provided under a collaborative effort between the National Institutes of Health and the U.S. Department of Agriculture. Searching the database simply involves typing your search terms in the box and selecting "Search."

Biotechnology & Patents

Biotechnology is the application of technology to manufacture products that improve biological processes for the benefit of living organisms. In medicine, biotechnology is the basis for the development of pharmaceutical drugs, diagnostic and testing equipment, surgical implants, assisted living devices, and nearly every other tangible product that improves patient lives and outcomes.

A **patent** is a form of **intellectual property**. Intellectual property is distinct from tangible property and refers to creations of the mind. Just as physical property rights protect a person from encroachment on tangle items, intellectual property rights protect a person from encroachment of creations of the mind. Intellectual property is generally divided into two categories, industrial property and copyright. Most often copyright applies to artistic works, like song lyrics, music scores, poems, novels, artistic paintings, photographs, and sculptures. Industrial property includes trademarks, industrial design, and patents and generally apply to physical items that are of utility for human use. Industrial property includes the ideas, thought, and reason that form the basis of an invention and are commonly expressed in mathematical calculations, engineering design, and the manipulation and combination of chemical processes and properties.

Most biotechnological creations are protected by patents. Most often intellectual property rights are asserted to prohibit **another** party from using creations of the mind in their own profit-making ventures. In addition to patents and copyright, two other common types of intellectual property are trademark and trade secrets. It is important to remember that intellectual property rights do **not** imply ownership, but rather the right to control the commercialization of the ideas or expression in question.

Patents can be an excellent source of information about not only patented drugs and medical devices but about disease and health conditions in general. Since patents are organized in a uniform and consistent manner, the introduction or background section can provide an excellent review of current scientific literature about a disease and also detailed discussions about various health care topics.

While property rights to physical items establish exclusive ownership rights to property that can be seen and felt, intellectual property rights establish ownership rights to creations of the mind. Besides patents, copyright and trademarks are the most the common types of intellectual property. According to the U.S. Patent and Trademark Office: "a patent is an intellectual property right granted by the Government of the United States of America to an inventor 'to exclude others from making, using, offering for sale, or selling the invention throughout the United States or importing the invention into the United States' for a limited time in exchange for public disclosure of the invention when the patent is granted." ("USPTO Glossary," n.d.)

Since patent applications are filed as long as five years before patent approval, these filings can give the researcher a glimpse into the future of the treatment, and sometimes even cures, for various diseases and health conditions.

While three types of patents can be granted, the two most common patents related to health care are **Utility Patents** and **Design Patents**. Utility patents protect inventions and discoveries of useful and new processes, machines, articles of manufacture, or "compositions of matter." As the name implies, design patents protect the drawings, charts, etc. that establish the shape and physical characteristics of an object to be manufactured. The third type of patent is the **Plant Patent** and is reserved for the discovery or invention of a new variety of "asexually" reproduced plant. Again, plant patents are uncommon in biotechnology.

Patent Information Online

The two most popular sources for patents granted in the United States are Google Patents https://www.google.com/patents and the U.S. Patent and Trademark Office by using either the quick search option http://patft.uspto.gov/netahtml/PTO/search-bool.html or the advanced search option http://patft.uspto.gov/netahtml/PTO/search-adv.htm.

The quick search option enables researchers to search up to two (2) research terms and also allows search results to be limited to specific fields or parts of the patent including applicant name and issue date.

Clinical Guidelines

As the name implies, a clinical guideline is a document that outlines the clinical management of a disease or health condition. In this regard, a clinical guideline can be viewed as a blueprint for the doctor and health care team to follow to diagnosis, manage, and treat specific health conditions in patients. Like any blueprint, however, the doctor must also incorporate her knowledge, experience, and best professional judgment and alter her application of a clinical guideline by taking into consideration the particular physical and emotional state of the patient, as well as the patients set of values and beliefs. Therefore, in practice the use of clinical guidelines by physicians is just that, a guideline used in conjunction with several other considerations to determine patient care.

Clinical guidelines generally cover every aspect of patient care, from diagnosis to treatment and prognosis and continuing care. The clinical guideline will typically also outline the risks and benefits of a course of action, as well as cost-effectiveness.

An important societal objective of clinical guidelines is to standardize medical care; thereby allowing patients regardless of income or socioeconomic status to receive the same high quality medical care.

Agency for Healthcare Research and Quality (AHRQ)

Clinical guidelines are generally collected and approved, and frequently written by a national health care agency. In the United States, the U.S. Agency for Healthcare Research and Quality (AHRQ) acts as the clearinghouse for clinical guidelines even though many are written by professional medical and doctor and associations. The AHRQ collection of guidelines can be accessed at http://www.guideline.gov/. Searching clinical guidelines at AHRQ is easy as the site uses similar syntax as a normal web search. Thus, to find a guideline for treating a specific disease simply enter your term in the search box. Likewise, to search for guidelines for conditions containing multiple words or phrases, enclose your terms in quotation marks. Finally, boolean searches can be performed using "and" or "or" between words and concepts of interest.

Drugs & Medications

Drugs are chemical substances that have a biological effect on humans and animals. Drugs are used by physicians to treat, cure, prevent, and even diagnose disease. Additionally, drugs can be used to enhance or improve mental or physical or well-being. Both prescription and over-the-counter drugs play several important roles in medicine. Drugs used to prevent disease are known as **Prophylactic Drugs**, drugs used to relieve symptoms are called **Palliative Drugs** and drugs used to cure disease are **Therapeutic Drugs**. Drugs for these purposes are also called medications or medicine, thus distinguishing them from drugs used for recreational or illicit purposes.

While all approved drugs have specific medicinal properties, most also have side effects. Side effects are secondary effects of medication that generally have no therapeutic value in the cure, treatment, or prevention of disease. Side effects can be both good and bad, but are most often the latter. One major challenge drug manufacturers face is developing medications that maximize the therapeutic effects of a drug while minimizing side effects.

When prescribing medications or recommending over-the-counter alternatives, doctors consider both the "good" and the "bad" when determining the best course of medicinal treatment for patients.

Prescription and Over-the-Counter Drugs and Medications

The best single resource to research drugs and medications is the **Drug Information Portal** administered by the National Institutes of Health (NIH). Unlike a standard web database, a portal is a site that functions as a point of access to multiple search engines or databases on the Internet. The NIH Drug Information Portal simultaneously searches for summary and detailed information across a number of federal government drug databases. While the number of actual sources returned varies depending on the drug searched, each drug term entered will be searched in the following databases:

Databases Providing Summary Information:

- Drug information (MedlinePlusDrug)
-
    - http://www.nlm.nih.gov/medlineplus/druginformation.html
- Dietary supplements and herbs (MedlinePlusSupp)
-
    - http://www.nlm.nih.gov/medlineplus/druginfo/herb_All.html
- Consumer health information (MedlinePlusTopics)
-
    - http://www.nlm.nih.gov/medlineplus/
- HIV/AIDS treatment (AIDSinfo)
-
    - http://www.aidsinfo.nih.gov/
- Breastfeeding (LactMed)
-
    - http://toxnet.nlm.nih.gov/newtoxnet/lactmed.htm
- Drug-Induced Liver Injury (LiverTox)
-
    - http://livertox.nih.gov/
- Drug labels (DailyMed)
-

- http://dailymed.nlm.nih.gov/
- Ingredients found in dietary supplements (Dietary Supplements Labels Database)
  - http://www.dsld.nlm.nih.gov/dsld/
- Clinical trials (ClinicalTrials.gov)
  - https://clinicaltrials.gov/
- Drug Identification with images (Pillbox beta)
  - http://pillbox.nlm.nih.gov/

Databases Providing Detailed Summary Information:

- Biological and physical data (HSDB)
  - http://toxnet.nlm.nih.gov/cgi-bin/sis/htmlgen?HSDB
- Scientific journals (Medline/PubMed)
  - http://www.ncbi.nlm.nih.gov/pubmed
- Toxicological journals (TOXLINE)
  - http://toxnet.nlm.nih.gov/cgi-bin/sis/htmlgen?TOXLINE
- Biological and chemical structures (PubChem)
  - https://pubchem.ncbi.nlm.nih.gov/
- Biological components of viruses (NIAID ChemDB)
  - http://chemdb.niaid.nih.gov/
- Toxicology and chemical components (ChemIDplus)
  - http://chem.sis.nlm.nih.gov/chemidplus/

Additional Drug Information Resources

- U.S. Food & Drug Administration (Drugs@FDA)
  - http://www.accessdata.fda.gov/scripts/cder/drugsatfda/

- U.S. Drug Enforcement Administration (DEA)
-
    - http://www.deadiversion.usdoj.gov/
- U.S. government search engine for all government resources (USA.gov)
-
    - http://www.usa.gov/

Information on more than 49,000 drugs and medications is included in the portal and drugs can be searched by either drug name or drug category (anticonvulsants, antidepressants, hallucinogens, etc.). The Drug Information portal is located at: http://druginfo.nlm.nih.gov/drugportal/drugportal.jsp

Books

Books can be an excellent source of medical information about Whiplash. Typically, the best books can provide the researcher with both excellent background information and wide-ranging (but less in-depth) treatment about a health condition or disease. Books are best when you need a broad overview about a health condition, or you want to learn a "little about a lot" of topics associated with a disease or disorder. Books are also appropriate when you don't need timely or cutting-edge information about a health condition. In this regard, books are best for well-established health conditions, with a substantial and long-term history of general consensus regarding diagnosis, cause, treatment, and management protocols.

There are several reasons that books may be of limited utility for research purposes. First, the time between researching and writing a book to book publication and public availability can be a lengthy one. As such, for new health conditions, or those with evolving or ever-changing diagnostic standards or treatment protocols books may not be the best research option. Also, given the intense competition for readers, and space on the local bookstore shelves, books are necessarily broad-based to appeal to as many prospective readers as possible, and seldom address (or adequately address) obscure health conditions or narrow topics within a disease sufficiently.

While large retailers, like Amazon, Barnes and Noble, and WalMart may be excellent places to *purchase* books, they are not necessarily the best sources to *choose* which books contain the most authoritative and reliable information about Whiplash, regardless of whether the book is a recent "best seller" or achieves positive reader reviews. Suffice to say, numerous media reports have documented the ease by which authors and publishers are able to artificially inflate book sales and accumulate glowing book buyer reviews.

National Library of Medicine's Bookshelf

The National Library of Medicine (NLM) Bookshelf provides anyone free access to book citations and other documents of interest for researching topics in health, medicine, and other life sciences. Bookshelf allows users to browse general topics or search for specific information about health conditions and disease in thousands of high-quality, well-researched books. Some books listed here even allow the researcher to read a portion or the entire contents of a book or document online.

To access Bookshelf, simply go to http://www.ncbi.nlm.nih.gov/books and begin your research by either browsing or searching for available titles. The interface is user friendly and allows the reader to browse by subjects including Health Care, Evidence-based Medicine, Health Policy, Comparative Effectiveness Research, and Public Health. Additional filters are also available to search by Book, Report, Collection, Documentation, or Database.

Below are a number of authoritative book and document titles related to Whiplash.

Journals

Scholarly or academic health journals are different from the popular magazines you see in your supermarket or book store in a number of ways. Overall, while popular magazines are published to entertain a wide audience, academic health journals are written to advance the knowledge in a particular health related field. Other important differences between scholarly or academic journals and consumer magazines include:

1. Scholarly health journals publish **in-depth** articles by **experts** including **original** findings by the researcher who is also the article author. Popular magazines publish **general** information about someone else's

findings.

2. Scholarly health journals take care to provide complete author **credentials** to demonstrate the author's subject-matter expertise. Popular magazine authors are almost **professional writers** with no subject matter expertise.

3. Scholarly health journals use **specialized terminologies** with very specific meanings. Popular magazine are taught to use only words and terms that a typical 7th grade reader can understand to make sure articles appeal to a broad readership.

4. Scholarly health journals are typically read only by other **scholars**, **researchers**, and **students** in the health care field. Popular magazines are read by the **general public**, most of whom will have no particular expertise, interest, or background in health care.

5. Scholarly health journals make prominent use of **graphs**, **tables**, and **charts**. Popular magazines include glossy **graphics** and **photographs**, along with significant **advertising**.

6. Scholarly health journal articles follow are very specific **format** and **layout**. Popular magazine format is generally **informal**.

7. Scholarly health journal articles include many carefully chosen **references**. Popular magazines seldom use references and instead use seemingly random **quotations** by experts and others.

8. Scholarly health journal articles are **peer-reviewed** by other subject-matter experts to ensure accuracy. Popular magazines are **edited** by editors with no subject-matter expertise.

The following section instructs you on how to find the most important journals related to Whiplash and also lists the most important titles for further review.

MEDLINE Journals - The Abridged Index Medicus (AIM)

The National Institutes of Health (NIH), National Library of Medicine (NLM) MEDLINE and PubMed research databases currently provide anyone with internet access to citations for over 5,600 journal titles. The Abridged Index Medicus (AIM) was created to assist researchers by limiting the vast NLM holdings to a manageable number of important or "core" journals. AIM is provided by the NLM to "afford rapid access to selected biomedical journal literature of immediate interest to the practicing physician" and therefore, in the opinion of NLM researchers, represents the most important medical journals for the broadest numbers of physicians. AIM is available online as a subset of PubMed by limiting searches to "Core clinical journals." The complete current list of AIM core journals can be found by going to http://www.nlm.nih.gov/bsd/aim.html.

All MEDLINE Journals

Using PubMed, it is easy to find the journals related to the specific medical conditions, disorders, or issues important to you. Like any database, however, there are specific search strategies that will make retrieving information easier.

Current Journals

Due to the large number of journals currently indexed in MEDLINE, it is seldom feasible to print out the entire list. However, if you do want to view and save the entire updated list there are two primary methods.

For current titles indexed by MEDLINE go to the "NLM Catalog" at: http://www.ncbi.nlm.nih.gov/nlmcatalog and in the search box enter the term: **currentlyindexed** then click search.

A second method is to type **all [sb]** in the search box. Once the results appear go to the **"Journal subsets filter"** on the left sidebar of the page and **"More..."**

The selection will then expand as a pop-up box will display **"Journal subsets"**. Make sure only the box entitled **"Currently indexed in MEDLINE"** is selected and go to the bottom of the popup and click the blue **"Show"** button.

While nothing appears to happen you will now see the **"Currently indexed in MEDLINE"** filter the Journal Subsets list on located on the sidebar. Click the **"x"** in the popup to close it and then click on **"Currently indexed in MEDLINE"** filter in the left sidebar. This will rerun the search and return all journals currently indexed in MEDLINE.

In 2014, this search returned 5,663 unique journal titles currently indexed in the NLM catalog.

To save a copy of the search results, find the hyperlink entitled **"Send to:"** located near the top of the search page and just left of the sidebar on the right. From there you can choose to send as an email, save to a temporary clipboard, or save as text document.

If ever you need to start over, you can delete all filters by simply clicking **"clear"** located just to the right of **"Journal subsets"** in the left sidebar.

Current and Previously Indexed Journals

For journals that were once indexed by MEDLINE but are no longer indexed **and** journals currently indexed the search protocol is almost identical to the search for **All Current Journals**, except for minor changes in the search term or filter, depending on which you method you use.

Again, go to the "NLM Catalog" at: http://www.ncbi.nlm.nih.gov/nlmcatalog and in the search box enter the term: **reportedmedline** then click search.

A second method is to type **all [sb]** in the search box and then click search. Once the results appear go to the **"Journal subsets filter"** on the left sidebar of the page and **"More..."**

The selection will then expand as a pop-up box and display **"Journal subsets"**. This time make sure only the box entitled **"Journals currently or previously indexed in MEDLINE."** is selected and go to the bottom of the popup and click the blue **"Show"** button.

Again, while nothing appears to happen you will now see that the **"Journals currently or previously indexed in MEDLINE"** filter is active in the

Journal Subsets filter list. Click the close icon, marked as "**X**", in the popup to close it and then click on "**Journals currently or previously indexed in MEDLINE**" filter in the left sidebar. This will rerun the search and return all journals both formerly and currently indexed in MEDLINE.

In 2014, this search returned 14,804 unique journal titles both currently and previously indexed in the NLM catalog.

To save a copy of the search results, find the hyperlink entitled "**Send to:**" located near the top of the page, and just left of the right sidebar. From there you can choose to send the complete list as an email, save to a temporary clipboard, or save as a text document.

If ever you need to start over, you can delete all filters by simply clicking "**clear**" located just to the right of "**Journal subsets**" in the left sidebar.

To find journals related to Whiplash go to the NLM **Broad Subject Terms for Indexed Journals** web page at http://wwwcf.nlm.nih.gov/serials/journals/index.cfm. Arranged alphabetically, this is the MEDLINE catalog page for all journals related to specific diseases, disorders, and conditions and other medical issues. Simple select the letter [*correct letter here*] and scroll to and click Whiplash and a list of relevant journals will display.

To save a copy of the search results, again find the hyperlink entitled "**Send to:**" located near the top of the page and just left of the right sidebar. From there you can choose to send as an email, save to a temporary clipboard, or save as text document.

Using Filters to Search

Given the enormous amount of information stored by the NLM, the use of database filters is important to narrow your search to only relevant information. In the previous section, the use of the "**Currently indexed in MEDLINE**" and "**Journals currently or previously indexed in MEDLINE**" were explained but there are several other useful filters to help focus your research.

Use the NLM **Catalog filters** to collect dental, consumer health, or other journal subset lists:

First, retrieve all items in the **NLM Catalog** http://www.ncbi.nlm.nih.gov/nlmcatalog/ homepage and enter all [sb] in the search box.

In the Filters sidebar located on the Results page, click on **Currently indexed in MEDLINE**. If you require a different subset, instead of selecting **"Currently indexed in MEDLINE"**, click **"More"** and additional filtering options will display in a pop-up. The available filters allow you to construct subsets from the following journal categories:

- **Journals in electronic-only format**
- **Journals indexed from the electronic version**
- **Consumer Health journals**
- **Core clinical journals (AIM)**
- **Dental journals**
- **Index Medicus journals (IM)**
- **Nursing journals**
- **Additional subsets in the journal subset lists include:**
- **Referenced in NCBI DBs**
- **Only PubMed journals**
- **Currently indexed in MEDLINE**
- **Journals currently or previously indexed in MEDLINE**
- **PubMed Central journals**

- **PubMed Central forthcoming journals**

Check the box next to the filter you need and click the **"Show"** button. The selected filter will now be visible on the sidebar filter. Close the pop-up box and click the filter on the sidebar. This will re-run your search limiting the results to the filter you selected.

Journal Articles

In this last chapter we identified methods for finding the most important journals **titles** related to Whiplash. This chapter expands on this information by identifying the best methods to search for **articles** in these journal titles and other academic health publications. During the course of your review, remember that unlike popular magazines academic journals are written and structured in a very standard and formal manner. While you may consider the format or structure bland and unappealing, remember the fundamental purpose of journal articles is to impart knowledge and communicate information and not to entertain. In this regard, it is this structured and nondescript presentation of information that lends itself particularly well to communicating important medical information.

Journal articles are a primary research resource. They are typically narrowly-focused and are the best literature resource for high quality and concentrated treatment of a topic. Scholarly articles are written by experts, incorporate complex data and statistics, and often times are used to present the most important and cutting-edge information about the recognition and treatment of disease and health conditions. Furthermore, scholarly journals are peer-reviewed meaning they are not only written by experts but are also carefully and critically reviewed by other experts before publication.

Academic and scholarly health journal articles are the best resources for very recent information about a health disease or disorder and for narrow topics within the larger context of a health condition.

Types of Research Articles

Most medical journal articles fall into one of two article categories: basic biomedical research or clinical research.

Biomedical research is the study of how living beings function. Human bodies are composed of smaller living systems that have their own unique life cycles. Similarly, disease has a life cycle and how that cycle functions in the human body is the subject of many research papers. Basic research in biomedical sciences may investigate the way basic protein sequences work in living things. Biomedical research can explain how cells appear, replicate, communicate, function, die, and then disappear. Biomedical research is important because the processes studied can effect disease or ensure good health. Biomedical research seeks to define biological processes and to understand learn how the body functions when disease is present and when disease is absent. Research leading to the understanding of these processes results in the development of drugs and other therapies that can disrupt disease mechanisms and restore the body to good health. Often, biomedical research use insect, fish, or animal test subjects in place of humans.

Clinical research is a the branch of medical science that explores the safety and effectiveness of medical devices, diagnostic tests, and drug and other medical treatments intended for human use. Clinical research can be subdivided into three different types. The first is **patient-oriented research**. Patient-oriented research is conducted with human subjects. Unlike Biomedical research, the scientists interact directly with the people involved in the study. A variety of reasons may be given to use patient-oriented research such as investigating human disease mechanisms, therapeutic interventions, clinical trials and/or development of new technologies. A second class of clinical research is **epidemiology**. "Epidemiology is the study of the distribution and determinants of health-related states or events (including disease), and the application of this study to the control of diseases and other health problems." ("Epidemiology," n.d.)

The final type of clinical research is **behavioral studies**. Behavioral studies focus on the actions, behaviors, and responses of individuals, groups, or species in its natural environment. The way a living being reacts to stimulation in regards to action and response is considered behavior. Behavior scientists studies are conducted on both humans and other animals and seek descriptions, generalizations, and explanations of behavior.

Clinical research can also be performed in the fields of physiology, pathophysiology, mental health and health services, education, and outcomes but are less common than the types of research discussed above.

The National Library of Medicine

This section focuses on the three most popular health-research databases, all administered by the National Institutes of Health (NIH), National Library of Medicine. These databases were chosen for several reasons. First, the NIH databases contain the most comprehensive and respected collection of academic and professional journal reference information available today. Second, the NIH databases are free to anyone with an Internet connection. While other excellent databases do exist, most simply "interface" with the NIH databases and can cost several hundreds, or even thousands of dollars a month to access.

The singular mission of the NIH is to perform original scientific biomedical and health research. As mentioned earlier, NIH researchers in the **Intramural Research Program (IRP)** perform in-house research and professionals in the **Extramural Research Program (ERP)** provide funding for research performed by scientists in academic institutions and other scientific research organizations. In 2013, 8,000 research grants were awarded funding out of nearly 50,000 applications received. Each year, approximately one-fourth of all scientific health research in the United States is fund by the NIH.

The NIH, National Library of Medicine (NLM) is the world's largest health research and biomedical library. Among its on-site holdings are more than 7 million medical-related books, journals, manuscripts, transcripts, and medical images. Perhaps even more impressive, is the NLM's online databases, search engine, and tools that allow scientists and the general public worldwide to access vital health-related information, including journal articles and data, and perform important medical research.

National Library of Medicine Databases

The three major information resources provided by the NLM are **MEDLINE, PubMed, and PubMed Central.**

MEDLINE

MEDLINE is comprised of scholary journal citations (including abstracts) for life science published in the U.S. and internationally. MEDLINE contains citations for approximately 5,400 biomedical journals published in the United States and worldwide. Coverage includes more than 21 million citations dating back to 1946. The MEDLINE database includes citations and abstracts in the fields of medicine, nursing, dentistry, veterinary medicine, health care systems and pre-clinical sciences to be offered through PubMed.

PubMed

PubMed consists of nearly 24 million citations for health science literature found in MEDLINE, books, and academic journals. Journal article citations link directly full-text articles and papers in PubMed Central and to publisher sites for articles not archived in PubMed Central. PubMed is free resource and available throughout the world.

PubMed Central

PubMed Central is a vast archive of medical and life science journal literature. Notably, all literature in PubMed Central is full-text meaning anyone can access the some of most important medical research conducted throughout the world.

PubMed Journal Citations

To begin using searching strategies outlined above enter your search term at the PubMed search link below.

http://www.ncbi.nlm.nih.gov/pubmed/

PubMed Central (PMC) Journal Citations

PubMed Central can be searched within PubMed or by going directly to the PubMed Central search link at:

http://www.ncbi.nlm.nih.gov/pmc/

Printed in Great Britain
by Amazon